Depression in Primary Care
Evidence and Practice

Depression in Primary Care

Evidence and Practice

Edited by

Simon Gilbody

Peter Bower

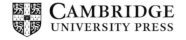

CAMBRIDGE
UNIVERSITY PRESS

CAMBRIDGE UNIVERSITY PRESS
Cambridge, New York, Melbourne, Madrid, Cape Town, Singapore,
São Paulo, Delhi, Dubai, Tokyo, Mexico City

Cambridge University Press
The Edinburgh Building, Cambridge CB2 8RU, UK

Published in the United States of America by Cambridge University Press, New York

www.cambridge.org
Information on this title: www.cambridge.org/9780521870504

© Cambridge University Press 2011

First published 2011

Printed in the United Kingdom at the University Press, Cambridge

A catalogue record for this publication is available from the British Library

Library of Congress Cataloguing in Publication data
Depression in primary care : evidence and practice / [edited by] Simon Gilbody, Peter Bower.
    p. ; cm.
Includes bibliographical references and index.
ISBN 978-0-521-87050-4 (pbk.)
1. Primary care (Medicine) 2. Depression, Mental. I. Gilbody, Simon M.
II. Bower, Peter (Peter J.)
[DNLM: 1. Depressive Disorder–therapy. 2. Primary Health Care–methods.
3. Quality Assurance, Health Care–methods. WM 171]
RC537.D43835 2011
616.85′27–dc22
2010028674

ISBN 978-0-521-87050-4 Paperback

Simon Gilbody: To Cathy and the joyful chaos that is the Gilbody brood.

Peter Bower: To Luke and Nicki, for taking me away from all this.

Contents

Notes on contributors

Simon Gilbody

Simon Gilbody is Professor of Psychological Medicine and Health Services Research at the University of York and Hull-York Medical School. He conducts reviews and clinical trials in primary care mental health, and is an honorary consultant in Primary Care Psychiatry. Simon is a longstanding contributor and editor within the Cochrane Collaboration.

Peter Bower

Peter Bower is Reader in Health Services Research at the Health Sciences Research Group, University of Manchester, and the National Institute for Health Research National School for Primary Care Research. He has a longstanding interest in the effectiveness of mental health treatments and in outcomes research.

John Cape

John Cape is Head of Psychology, Camden and Islington NHS Foundation Trust, and Visiting Professor, Division of Psychology and Language Sciences, University College London. He has a longstanding research interest in mental health in primary care and in the organization of mental health services between primary and secondary care.

Craig Whittington

Since 2001, Craig has worked as the Senior Systematic Reviewer for the National Collaborating Centre for Mental Health, based at the British Psychological Society Centre for Outcomes Research and Effectiveness, University College London.

David Richards

David Richards is Professor of Mental Health Services Research at Exeter University's Mood Disorders Centre. He has been extensively involved in the

Improving Access to Psychological Therapies programme, and runs a multi-centre research team funded by the Medical Research Council and the National Institute for Health Research, which develops and tests new models of delivering treatment.

Stephen Thielke

Stephen Thielke is Assistant Professor in the Department of Psychiatry and Behavioral Sciences at the University of Washington and a researcher in the Geriatric Research, Education, and Clinical Center of the Puget Sound VA. His research focuses on health and healthcare utilization during ageing. He is developing predictive models for depression to help with the assessment, longitudinal monitoring, and treatment of mental health symptoms in older adults.

Jürgen Unützer

Jürgen Unützer is Professor and Vice-Chair of Psychiatry at the University of Washington and an affiliate investigator at the Group Health Research Institute. A geriatric psychiatrist and health services researcher, Jürgen was the principal investigator of project IMPACT, a multisite study to improve care for late-life depression funded by the John A Hartford Foundation and the California HealthCare Foundation. As director of the AIMS Center focused on Advancing Integrated Mental Health Solutions, he has helped implement evidence-based collaborative care for depression and other common mental disorders in over 500 primary care clinics in the United States and several other countries.

Preface

We both have a bit of a reputation as systematic reviewers, and a glance down our CVs means that we are guilty as charged. Frankly, it is not always the best reputation to have. Systematic reviews are sometimes seen as largely technical in nature, ignoring the complex and messy reality of healthcare delivery and reducing everything to a few calculations and a pretty graph. They are also seen as the preserve of methodologically and statistically minded types, the sort of people who are excessively concerned with minutiae and routinely miss the wood while comprehensively searching for the best concealed trees.

Part of the reason for creating this book was to show that reviews can be more than that – that it is possible to link the review process with complex policy issues, and to use the insights generated from reviews to assist in decision making in ways that go beyond simple statements about this or that being effective at such and such a level of significance. However, we also wanted to share our enthusiasm for reviews, because they are actually quite simple and potentially accessible to a wide range of people, and because they remain a crucial part of the scientific armoury and will only get more important as the amount, scope and complexity of research increases.

This book is not meant to provide an answer to the problems of delivering services for depression. The area is too complex, and too value-laden, to submit to such a straightforward approach. What we aim to do is show how the techniques of systematic review and evidence synthesis can be used to make sense of a large and complex literature, to challenge assumptions and provide fresh insights, and add to the debate about the best way to help patients in need. Although the aspiration of the systematic review enterprise is somehow to create a process that would lead to the same result, no matter who did the review, that will only ever remain an aspiration. Ambiguity and subjectivity have a way of creeping into the process, so that the final result is always up for debate. But it is precisely within those debates where the useful work begins.

We would like to acknowledge the many academic and clinical colleagues who have contributed to this endeavour. Some have contributed directly as authors, but we would also like to thank all those colleagues who have shaped our thinking about mental health research and service delivery over the years, and have thus contributed in a more roundabout way. Multidisciplinary research being what it is, there are simply too many to name you all, but special thanks (in appropriately random order) go to Karina Lovell, Martin Roland, Linda Gask, Bonnie Sibbald, Anne Rogers, Michael King, Michael Barkham, Robert West, Andre Tylee, Rachel Churchill, Allan House, Trevor Sheldon, David Richards and David Torgerson.

We would also like to take the chance to acknowledge the support and patience of Nisha Doshi of Cambridge University Press and her help in completing this project. We realise that we were better at setting deadlines than meeting them, but we hope the final product makes the frustrations you faced along the way worthwhile.

Depression in primary care

Simon Gilbody

Case study

Jean is a 58-year-old woman who has worked as a teacher for 26 years. She comes to the primary care practice to see Dr Stevens. Her daughter is concerned that her mother is 'under a lot of stress and is not coping'. Jean expresses feelings of frustration, a short temper and lack of purpose in her home, family and work life. She has two late-teenage children, one of whom has recently left home. She works hard in her job as a teacher at a local school. She married in her early twenties and her husband is inattentive and drinks excessively.

During her consultation she appears tearful, shrunken and afraid. She describes a range of physical and psychological symptoms including tiredness, poor concentration and lack of motivation. Her appetite is poor and she has stopped cooking for herself and the family. She feels negative about the future but has no plans to end her own life. She has found it difficult to get to work in the past month and wants a sick note to allow her a week or two to get on top of things.

The case study outlined above will be familiar to many healthcare professionals and to a significant proportion of their patients. Depression is a very common mental health problem and is associated with a great deal of personal suffering, as well as acting as a significant burden on health services.

Managing depression effectively is a major challenge, and one that has exercised patients, professionals and policy makers worldwide. There is increasing consensus that the best place to treat depression is in primary care. For example, the recent World Health Organization report *Integrating mental health into primary care: a global perspective*[1] stated seven reasons why treatment for mental health problems such as depression should be based in primary care (Box 1.1).

The principles outlined by the World Health Organization in Box 1.1 seem reasonable and consistent. But recent years have seen changes to the way in which health policy is made and evaluated, away from ideology and aspiration

Depression in Primary Care: Evidence and Practice, ed. Simon Gilbody and Peter Bower. Published by Cambridge University Press. © Cambridge University Press 2011.

Box 1.1 Reasons for treating mental health in primary care[1]

1. **The burden of mental disorders is great**. Mental disorders are prevalent in all societies. They create a substantial personal burden for affected individuals and their families, and they produce significant economic and social hardships that affect society as a whole.
2. **Mental and physical health problems are interwoven**. Many people suffer from both physical and mental health problems. Integrated primary care services help ensure that people are treated in a holistic manner, meeting the mental health needs of people with physical disorders, as well as the physical health needs of people with mental disorders.
3. **The treatment gap for mental disorders is enormous**. In all countries, there is a significant gap between the prevalence of mental disorders, on the one hand, and the number of people receiving treatment and care, on the other hand. Primary care for mental health helps close this gap.
4. **Primary care for mental health enhances access**. When mental health is integrated into primary care, people can access mental health services closer to their homes, thus keeping their families together and maintaining their daily activities. Primary care for mental health also facilitates community outreach and mental health promotion, as well as long-term monitoring and management of affected individuals.
5. **Primary care for mental health promotes respect of human rights**. Mental health services delivered in primary care minimize stigma and discrimination. They also remove the risk of human rights violations that can occur in psychiatric hospitals.
6. **Primary care for mental health is affordable and cost effective**. Primary care services for mental health are less expensive than psychiatric hospitals, for patients, communities and governments alike. In addition, patients and families avoid indirect costs associated with seeking specialist care in distant locations. Treatment of common mental disorders is cost effective, and investments by governments can bring important benefits.
7. **Primary care for mental health generates good health outcomes**. The majority of people with mental disorders treated in primary care have good outcomes, particularly when linked to a network of services at secondary level and in the community.

and towards the use of objective and transparent forms of knowledge. This has often been identified with a movement called 'evidence-based practice'. This was succinctly summarized by one of its originators in medicine, who defined it as 'the conscientious, explicit, and judicious use of current best evidence in making decisions'.[2] Box 1.2 presents a full definition of evidence-based practice in the context of medicine.

Evidence-based practice changes according to context. The evidence-based practice of a clinician deciding on a treatment for an individual patient will differ

Box 1.2 The definition of evidence-based medicine[2]

Evidence-based medicine is the conscientious, explicit and judicious use of current best evidence in making decisions about the care of individual patients. The practice of evidence-based medicine means integrating individual clinical expertise with the best available external clinical evidence from systematic research. By individual clinical expertise we mean the proficiency and judgement that individual clinicians acquire through clinical experience and clinical practice. Increased expertise is reflected in many ways, but especially in more effective and efficient diagnosis and in the more thoughtful identification and compassionate use of individual patients' predicaments, rights and preferences in making clinical decisions about their care. By best available external clinical evidence we mean clinically relevant research, often from the basic sciences of medicine, but especially from patient-centred clinical research into the accuracy and precision of diagnostic tests (including the clinical examination), the power of prognostic markers and the efficacy and safety of therapeutic, rehabilitative and preventive regimens. External clinical evidence both invalidates previously accepted diagnostic tests and treatments, and replaces them with new ones that are more powerful, more accurate, more efficacious and safer.

from that of a policy maker considering changes to the way services are delivered for a locality. However, in both cases it has the aim of informing that decision using high-quality scientific evidence.

This book applies those principles to the problem of depression. We start, in this chapter, by outlining the nature of primary care, the role of primary care in the management of depression and the different outcomes of that care. We then go on to outline different ways in which primary care services for depression can be organized (Chapter 2), and review the various scientific methods we can use to evaluate those services (Chapters 3 and 4). The aim is to apply those methods to give an evidence-based assessment of the best way to care for depression in primary care (Chapters 5, 6, 7, 8, 9), consider the challenges of implementing those findings (Chapters 10,11, 12) and highlight the research issues for the future (Chapter 13).

What is primary care and primary mental healthcare?

Primary care services are sometimes referred to as general practice, family practice or family medicine. The terms are not synonymous, but together they have a number of common elements that are critical to understanding their role in depression.

Primary healthcare was defined by the Alma Ata declaration as 'essential health care based on practical, scientifically sound and socially acceptable methods and technology made universally accessible to individuals and families in the community through their full participation and at a cost that the community and country can afford to maintain at every stage of their development in the spirit of self-reliance and self-determination' (www.who.int/hpr/NPH/docs/declaration_almaata.pdf).

According to the Institute of Medicine,[3] primary care is the 'provision of integrated, accessible healthcare services by clinicians who are accountable for addressing a large majority of personal health needs, developing a sustained partnership with patients, and practicing in the context of the family and community'.

Descriptions of the core content of primary care vary,[4,5] but key aspects include:

- first contact care, with direct patient access
- care characterized by patient-centredness (i.e. consistent with patient needs and preferences), family orientation and continuity (i.e. care over time from a single professional)
- a role in the coordination of care (i.e. coordinating care from multiple agencies)
- a 'gate-keeping' function, regulating access to specialist care (i.e. care from clinicians who focus on certain types of problem or organ systems).

The structure of healthcare systems throughout the world varies widely, and the degree to which particular systems can be characterized as 'primary care-led' varies between countries and over time.[4,5] Some primary care systems act as gate-keepers to specialist services (as in the UK), others provide free-market services in parallel to specialist services, while others function in a complex system containing both types of access (as in the USA). Services also vary according to whether they are free to patients at the point of care delivery; whether they are led by doctors or non-medical staff; and the degree to which they provide continuity of care. There is some evidence that the degree of primary care focus in a healthcare system (especially the 'gate-keeping' role) is a key driver of the cost effectiveness and efficiency of healthcare provision.[6]

Mental healthcare in primary care is defined as 'the provision of basic preventive and curative mental health care at the first point of contact of entry into the health care system'.[7] Usually this means that care is provided by a primary care clinician, such as a general practitioner or nurse, who can refer complex cases to a more specialized mental health professional. The World Health Organization ATLAS survey found that 96% of European countries reported identified mental health activity in primary care, and 62% reported training facilities.[7]

What is depression?

A distinction is often made between 'severe and long-term mental health disorders' (most often associated with schizophrenia), and 'common mental health disorders' (most often associated with anxiety and depression). Although primary care has an important role to play in the management of more severe disorders, recent policy in many healthcare systems has highlighted the role of specialist services in their management. 'Common' disorders are viewed as more appropriately within the remit of primary care, partly by default, as specialist services have refocused their energies, and partly by design, as primary care is seen as being able to provide appropriate, patient-centred care to this population.

'Common' disorders can be described using standard diagnostic classifications.[8] Box 1.3 shows the diagnostic criteria for depression used by the World Health Organization *International Classification of Diseases* (ICD-10) system and American Psychiatric Association *Diagnostic and Statistical Manual of Mental Disorders* (DSM-IV). Overlapping disorders may exist along a spectrum of anxiety, depression, somatization and substance misuse in primary care. Sub-threshold conditions (i.e. disorders not meeting full diagnostic criteria for mental disorders in DSM-IV or ICD-10) are prevalent and associated with significant costs and disability.[9] There remains significant controversy over the nature of depression and the adequacy of different systems for classifying and describing the phenomenon and distinguishing it from other problems and disorders.

Patients with long-term medical illness (particularly diabetes, coronary heart disease and stroke) have a high prevalence of major depressive illness.[12–15] Evidence suggests that both depressive symptoms and major depression may be associated with increased morbidity and mortality from such illnesses.[16]

A useful overview of the major environmental, social and interpersonal causes of depression is given by Gilbody and Gask.[17] Higher rates of attendance and treatment for depression are associated with socially disadvantaged populations: people living in deprived areas (especially the inner city but also deprived rural areas); people who are unemployed, and living on benefits; and victims of violence, either domestic violence or living in violent areas. Depression is also associated with a lack of social support, being more common among people who are divorced or separated; single parents (usually women); widowed elderly people; non-religious communities, and communities with fewer extended families, where people are more likely to be living alone. Women consult primary care professionals much more frequently than men, who, in the age range 20–45 years, rarely consult. Depression in primary care is often viewed in terms of the stress-vulnerability model,[18] which states that destabilization (getting symptoms) is the result of longlasting vulnerability factors (genetic risk, early life experience, physical illness and lack of social support) acting in concert with exposure to environmental stressors, usually one or more highly stressful events of which the most common are loss events (bereavement, loss of occupation, loss of health).

Outcomes of depression

Community-based epidemiological studies have confirmed that many people have recurrent or chronic depression,[19,20] but the risk of recurrence or chronicity in depressed primary care patients and the level of disability associated with this risk remain uncertain. There have been relatively few studies in this setting, and some of these studies have not collected repeated data throughout the follow-up period while others have relied on retrospective data.[21] However, what is beginning to emerge from the literature in this setting is a picture of major depression, in around 40–50% of those given the diagnosis, as a relapsing and remitting

Box 1.3 Diagnostic criteria for depressive disorders from the World Health Organization (WHO) ICD-10[10] and American Psychiatric Association DSM-IV[11]

	ICD 10 Depressive disorder	DSM-IV Major depressive disorder
Clinical significance	Some difficulty in continuing with ordinary work and social activities, but will probably not cease to function completely in mild depressive episode; considerable difficulty in continuing with social, work or domestic activities in moderate depressive episode; considerable distress or agitation, and unlikely to continue with social, work or domestic activities, except to a very limited extent in severe depressive episode	Symptoms cause clinically significant stress or impairment in social, occupational or other important areas of functioning
Duration of symptoms	A duration of at least 2 weeks is usually required for diagnosis for depressive episodes of all three grades of severity	Most of day, nearly every day for at least 2 weeks.
Severity	Depressed mood, loss of interest and enjoyment and reduced energy leading to increased fatigability and diminished activity in typical depressive episodes; other common symptoms are: (1) Reduced concentration and attention (2) Reduced self-esteem/self-confidence (3) Ideas of guilt and unworthiness (4) Bleak and pessimistic views of the future (5) Ideas or acts of self-harm or suicide (6) Disturbed sleep (7) Diminished appetite For **mild depressive episode**, 2 of most typical symptoms of depression and 2 of the other symptoms are required. 　For **moderate depressive episode**, 2 of 3 of most typical symptoms of depression and at least 3 of the other symptoms are required. 　For **severe depressive episode**, all 3 of the typical symptoms noted for mild and moderate depressive episodes are present and at least 4 other symptoms of severe intensity are required	Five or more of following symptoms; at least one symptom is either depressed mood or loss of interest or pleasure: (1) Depressed mood (2) Loss of interest (3) Significant weight loss or gain or decrease or increase in appetite (4) Insomnia or hypersomnia (5) Psychomotor agitation or retardation (6) Fatigue or loss of energy (7) Feelings of worthlessness or excessive or inappropriate guilt (8) Diminished ability to think or concentrate, or indecisiveness (9) Recurrent thoughts of death, recurrent suicidal ideation without a specific plan, or suicide attempt or a specific plan

condition. In a large World Health Organization study in primary care, depression emerged as a chronic disorder: one year after entry to the study, about 60% of those treated with medication, and 50% of the milder depressions, still met criteria for depression.[22]

Ronalds and colleagues[23] followed up patients in British general practice with a diagnosis of depression, anxiety or panic disorder for a period of six months. Good outcome was predicted by mild depression at initial assessment, high educational level and being in employment. At follow-up the most important predictor of improvement was reduction in marked difficulties over the six months. Recognition and management by the primary care professional was most frequent in patients with severe disorder, but such patients were least likely to improve because of the severity of their depression and marked social difficulties.

Costs of depression

The costs associated with depression in primary care arise in part due to increased consultation and the use of healthcare resources directly related to the management of depression. This is often compounded when depression goes unrecognized and patients present with physical rather than psychological symptoms.[24] Patients with depression also commonly have co-morbid physical disorders, and the presence of depression is associated with poor outcome of physical disorders and increased resource utiliztion,[12] including costly referrals to secondary care.[25] The economic burden of depression is also felt within society at large, through the burden that falls on carers and dependants, and through lost productivity and life years. The annual costs of depression are most commonly quoted from two studies as being US$83 billion in the USA[26] and £9 billion in the UK.[27]

Economists examine the burden of illness within 'cost of illness studies'[28] where the various costs associated with illness are estimated through a range of readily available data. These studies aim to estimate how much a society spends on a particular disorder, and where that money is spent. Cost of illness studies generally differentiate between 'direct', 'indirect' and 'intangible costs'. Direct costs include medical (e.g. outpatient, inpatient and pharmaceutical costs) and non-medical costs (e.g. transport and social services). Indirect costs include loss of productivity due to absence from the workplace or reduced productivity at the workplace caused by morbidity (morbidity costs) and premature death (mortality costs). Intangible costs result from the restriction of the quality of life of the sufferer and their families. Because an accurate quantification in monetary terms is difficult, they are often not considered in cost-of-illness studies.

A useful overview of this topic is presented by Luppa and colleagues.[29] They identified 24 studies from a range of healthcare settings (mostly the USA and Europe) and one major cross-national study from a range of European countries.[30] These studies measured the direct and indirect costs associated with depression. Using a variety of methods to provide some consistency and comparability between studies, they presented data on 'costs per depressed case' based on the reported prevalence data and costs per inhabitant.[31] The direct costs associated with depression ranged from US$244 to US$2488 per year. In terms of indirect costs, costs per case varied widely between countries and healthcare settings, namely from US$94 to US$5361. Differences resulted from inclusion of different costs (absenteeism from work, reduced capacity at the workplace, inclusion of housework) as well as from the value of the earnings used. Mortality costs per case were similar across countries (US$371 per year in the UK and between US$235 and US$388 per year in the USA).

These studies demonstrate that depression is associated with a substantial increase in costs, leading to a high economic burden. They have proved useful in raising the importance of depression within wider health, social and economic decision making: in the UK for example, the demonstration of the economic burden associated with depression has been instrumental in securing increased investment for depression services.[32] However, these studies give no direct guidance as to how depression should be managed in an effective and efficient way.

Depression in primary care: 'pathways to care'

A key to understanding how patients either receive or fail to receive the care they need comes from studying the epidemiology of common mental health problems and the flow of patients from the community through various healthcare settings. The most influential of these is the 'pathways to care' model first described by Goldberg and Huxley (Figure 1.1).[33,34]

The pathways to care model has five 'levels' and three 'filters'. Of all those individuals in the community, a high proportion consult their doctor in any one year, while a lesser number suffer an episode of mental ill health during the same time span. These patients pass the first filter ('the decision to consult'). Of those reaching the primary care services, a proportion of patients are recognized by the primary care clinician as suffering from disorder ('conspicuous psychiatric morbidity') and thus pass the second filter ('recognition by the primary care professional'). Passing the third and fourth filters involves referral to specialist mental health services or admission to a specialist hospital. Although there may be exceptions to this referral process, and variations depending on the local structure of services,[35] it provides an adequate general model for mental health in most primary care-led services.

Stigma within society and poor knowledge about the nature of mental health often prevents people from consulting with problems in the first instance.[33] For those who do consult, a wealth of evidence has indicated that recognition of disorders is less than optimal,[36,37] and that, furthermore, there is wide variation in recognition rates between primary care clinicians.[38] Patients who are recognized often do not receive quality of care in line with current guidelines, either in relation to pharmacological treatments or the provision of evidence-based non-pharmacological interventions.[39,40,41] Finally, provision of specialist services (such as psychological therapists working on-site in primary care) often varies widely.[42,43]

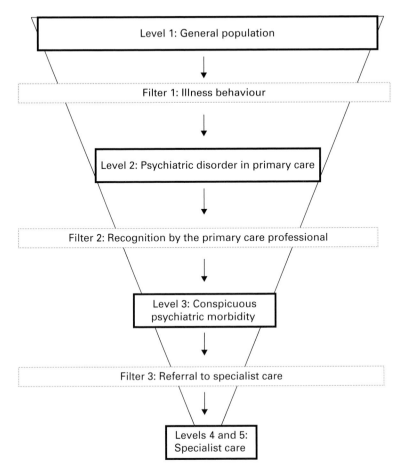

Figure 1.1 The pathways to care model.[33]

The presentation of depression in primary care

As we move from community settings to primary care settings, the prevalence of major depression increases from 3–5% to about 5–10%.[34,44]

Diagnosis is a less precise (and less frequent) activity in primary care than it is in specialist care. Primary care professionals are more likely to think in terms of problems than diagnoses. They are more likely to make a diagnosis of depression if they believe they can manage and treat it: diagnosis tends to follow management decisions, not precede them.[45] In the USA, primary care professionals are often trained to separate patients by level of severity of symptoms, and to carry out full mental health diagnostic assessment only for patients with significant or persistent symptoms.[46]

When compared with formal psychiatric diagnoses, depression frequently remains undetected and untreated,[47] because of co-morbidity with physical illness or presentation of physical symptoms by the patient. However, although this finding has led to considerable criticism of primary care workers, there is evidence that depression which is unrecognized by primary care workers is less severe[48] and has a more favourable outcome.[22]

Depression and the doctor–patient relationship in primary care

In a study of adults with a diagnosis of depression in primary care in the UK,[49] some exhibited an unquestioning attitude to quality of care for their problems. A recurring theme among those with depression was the sense of 'wasting the doctor's time', and a sense that it was not possible for doctors to listen to them and understand how they felt.

Khan and colleagues,[50] who primarily looked at experiences in the UK setting, noted that external sources of stress or conflict were drawn upon most frequently to account for the presence of depression. These included conflict with work colleagues or family, long-term conditions, events in childhood, material disadvantage and racism.[51–54] Rather than emphasizing symptoms or feelings of depression, personal experience of depression was characterized by expressions of being unable to cope, and in particular disturbances to everyday functioning and social roles.[55,56] Patients' descriptions of the cause of their problems notably differed from the psychological or biomedical explanations underlying conventional treatments such as psychological therapy and antidepressants.

Policy goals in primary care mental health

Previous sections have highlighted the prevalence of depression and the burden that accompanies it, and outlined the way in which depressed patients interact with primary care services. The potential role of primary care services should be clear. However, setting policies about how best to deliver primary care services requires a statement of goals (and priorities among goals), as well as a statement of the best way of achieving those goals.

In terms of overall goals, the World Health Organization[7,57] suggests that all mental health policies are anchored by four goals: access; equity; effectiveness; and efficiency.

- *Access*: Service provision should meet the need for services in the community, and the right to obtain treatment should depend on need for services, not ability to pay or geographical location. This is especially important in the case of depression with reference to Goldberg and Huxley's 'pathways to care' model. There are problems in access to care in primary care, related to the fact that people do not consult as a consequence of stigma or inadequate knowledge, and a significant proportion of disorders presenting in this setting are not recognized by the gate-keeping primary care clinician. Patients failing to pass the first 'filter to care' are unable to access effective care from health services.

- *Equity*: Mental healthcare resources should be distributed fairly across the population at large, so that patients with similar problems receive similar services (horizontal equity) and patients with more severe problems receive more care than those with minor problems (vertical equity). There are two main sources of inequity in current primary care mental health services, which relate to the wide variation in the ability of individual practitioners to recognize disorders, and inequity in the provision of specialist mental health services. In addition, it could also be argued that investment in mental health services is inequitable compared with other disease groups.

- *Effectiveness*: Mental health services should do what they are intended to do – improve health and mental wellbeing. Health may be defined in terms of health status, or broader definitions may involve wider function and quality of life, and not just the absence of disease.[58] Current management of mental health problems can involve the provision of ineffective treatments or those of unknown effectiveness (such as some forms of psychological therapy), or the ineffective delivery of effective treatments (such as inappropriate use of medication).

- *Efficiency*: Given that resources for any healthcare system are limited, they should be distributed in such a way as to maximize health gains to society. Clearly, the problems in access, equity and effectiveness identified above limit the degree to which current services can be efficient.

Policy makers are increasingly interested in a fifth goal:

- *Patient-centredness*: At a policy level, this relates to the degree to which services are 'closely congruent with, and responsive to patients' wants, needs and preferences'.[59] Current health policy aims to achieve this using a number of mechanisms, such as increasing patient choice, measuring satisfaction with care, and including patients in the design of services. In the UK, this has been summarized in recent policy documents as giving patients 'more choice and a louder voice'.[60] 'Patient-centred services' are highly relevant to primary care. The Alma Ata declaration defined primary care as 'socially acceptable' healthcare made available through the 'full participation' of patients and families, and primary care systems have long been characterized as being oriented to the needs of patients and families rather than technology.[4] Therefore, primary care has the greatest potential to provide 'patient-centred services' within the broader health economy.

The relationships between these different goals are complex, and satisfying the different goals is a challenge, especially as they can conflict. For example, there may be tensions between the goals of a population-level approach to planning care (highlighting access and equity), and the goals relating to the treatment of an individual patient (where effectiveness and patient-centredness are key). As we review the scientific evidence to judge 'what works' in primary care, we will pay reference to these health policy goals, and the degree to which they can be achieved for depression in primary care.

Concluding comments

Depression is a prevalent and costly disorder. It is costly in terms of the suffering experienced by individuals and costly to healthcare systems and wider society in terms of the economic burden and inappropriate use of resources. Practice and policy should be based on good evidence of what works and what represents the optimum use of limited healthcare resources. The purpose of this book is to produce an accessible summary of the clinical and economic evidence to ensure that the delivery of primary care mental health reflects this evidence.

REFERENCES

1 World Health Organization. *World Organization of Family Doctors. Integrating mental health into primary care: a global perspective.* Geneva: World Health Organization/ WONCA, 2008.

2 Sackett DL, Rosenberg WMC, Gray JAM, Haynes RB, Richardson WS. Evidence based medicine: what it is and what it isn't. *British Medical Journal* 1996;312:71–2.

3 Institute of Medicine. *Primary Care: America's Health in a New Era.* Washington DC: Institute of Medicine, 1996.

4 Starfield B. *Primary Care: Concept, Evaluation and Policy.* New York: Oxford University Press, 1992.

5 Fry J, Horder J. *Primary Health Care in an International Context.* Abingdon, UK: Wace Burgess, 1994.

6 Boerma W, de Jong F, Mulder P. *Health Care and General Practice Across Europe.* Utrecht: NIVEL, Netherlands Institute of Primary Health Care, 1993.

7 World Health Organization. *ATLAS – Mental Health Resources in the World 2001.* Geneva: World Health Organization, 2001.

8 Ustun T, Goldberg D, Cooper J, Simon G, Sartorius N. New classification for mental disorders with management guidelines for use in primary care: ICD-10 PHC chapter five. *British Journal of General Practice* 1995;45:211–15.

9 Piccinelli M, Rucci P, Ustun B, Simon G. Typologies of anxiety, depression and somatization symptoms among primary care attenders with no formal mental disorders. *Psychological Medicine* 2002;29:677–88.

10 World Health Organization. *International Statistical Classification of Diseases and Related Health Problems – 10th Revision.* Geneva: World Health Organization, 1990.

11 American Psychiatric Association. *Diagnostic and Statistical Manual – 4th Edition.* Washington, DC: American Psychiatric Association, 1994.

12 Katon W, Ciechanowski P. Impact of major depression on chronic medical illness. *Journal of Psychosomatic Research* 2002;53:859–63.

13 Anderson S, Freedland K, Clouse R, Lustman P. The prevalence of comorbid depression in adults with diabetes. *Diabetes Care* 2001;24:1069–77.

14 Hemingway H, Marmot M. Evidence based cardiology: psychosocial factors in the aetiology and prognosis of coronary heart disease: systematic review of prospective cohort studies. *British Medical Journal* 1999;318:1460.

15 Kotila M, Numminen H, Waltimo O, Kaste M. Depression after stroke results of the FINNSTROKE study. *Stroke* 1998; 29:368–72.

16 Katon W. Clinical and health services relationships between major depression, depressive symptoms, and general medical illness. *Biological Psychiatry* 2003;54:216–26.

17 Gilbody S, Gask L. Depressive disorders in primary care. In: Herrman H, Maj M, Sartorius N, editors. *Depressive Disorders: World Psychiatric Association Evidence and Experience Series.* Melbourne: World Psychiatric Association & Wiley-Blackwell, 2009.

18 Goldberg D, Huxley P. *Common Mental Disorders: A Biosocial Model.* London: Tavistock, 1992.

19 Kessler RC, Berglund P, Demler O, Jin R, Merikangas K, Walters E. Lifetime prevalence and age-of-onset distributions of DSM-IV disorders in the National Comorbidity Survey Replication. *Archives of General Psychiatry* 2005;62:593–602.

20 Judd L, Akiskal H, Maser J. A prospective 12-year study of subsyndromal and syndromal depressive symptoms in unipolar major depressive disorders. *Archives of General Psychiatry* 1998;55:694–700.

21 Vuorilehto M, Melartin T, Isometsa E. Depressive disorders in primary care: recurrent, chronic and co-morbid. *Psychological Medicine* 2005;35:673–82.

22 Goldberg D, Privett M, Ustun B, Simon G, Linden M. The effects of detection and treatment on the outcome of major depression in primary care: a naturalistic study in 15 cities. *British Journal of General Practice* 1998;48:1840–4.

23 Ronalds C, Creed F, Stone K, Webb S, Tomenson B. Outcome of anxiety and depressive disorders in primary care. *British Journal of Psychiatry* 1997;171:427–33.

24 Kirmayer L, Robbins M, Dworkind M, Yaffe MJ. Somatization and the recognition of depression and anxiety in primary care. *American Journal of Psychiatry* 1993:734–41.

25 Simon GE, Revicki D, Heiligenstein J, Grothaus L, VonKorff M, Katon W, Hylan T. Recovery from depression, work productivity, and health care costs among primary care patients. *General Hospital Psychiatry* 2000;22:153–62.

26 Greenberg PE, Kessler R, Birnbaum H *et al.* The economic burden of depression in the United States: how did it change between 1990 and 2000? *Journal of Clinical Psychiatry* 2003;64:1465–75.

27 Thomas C, Morris S. Cost of depression among adults in England in 2000. *British Journal of Psychiatry* 2003;183:514–19.

28 Drummond M, Sculpher M, Stoddard G, O'Brien B, Torrance G. *Methods for the Economic Evaluation of Health Care*, 3rd edn. Oxford: Oxford University Press, 2005.

29 Luppa M, Heinrich S, Matthias J *et al.* Cost-of-illness studies of depression: A systematic review. *Journal of Affective Disorders* 2007;98:29–43.

30 Chisholm D, Diehr P, Knapp M, Patrick D, Treglia M, Simon G. Depression status, medical comorbidity and resource costs. Evidence from an international study of major depression in primary care (LIDO). *British Journal of Psychiatry* 2003;183:121–31.

31 Organisation for Economic Co-operation and Development. *(OECD) Health Data, Statistics and Indicators for 30 Countries.* Geneva: OECD, 2005.

32 Layard R. *Mental Health: Britain's Biggest Social Problem?* London: Prime Minister's Strategy Unit, 2004.

33 Goldberg D, Huxley P. *Mental Illness in the Community.* London: Tavistock, 1980.

34 Gask L. Overt and covert barriers to the integration of primary and specialist mental health care. *Social Science and Medicine* 2005;61:1785–94.

35 Gater R, De Almeida e Sousa B, Barrientos G *et al.* The pathways to psychiatric care: a cross-cultural study. *Psychological Medicine* 1991;21:761–74.

36 Paykel E, Priest R. Recognition and management of depression in general practice: consensus statement. *British Medical Journal* 1992;305:1198–202.

37 Tiemens B, Ormel J, Simon G. Occurrence, recognition and outcome of psychological disorders in primary care. *American Journal of Psychiatry* 1996;153:636–44.

38 Marks J, Goldberg D, Hillier V. Determinants of the ability of general practitioners to detect psychiatric illness. *Psychological Medicine* 1979;9:337–53.

39 Katon W, von Korff M, Lin E, Bush T, Ormel J. Adequacy and duration of antidepressant treatment in primary care. *Medical Care* 1992;30:67–76.

40 Katon W, Von Korff M Lin E *et al.* Population-based care of depression: effective disease management strategies to decrease prevalence. *General Hospital Psychiatry* 1997;19:169–78.

41 Schulberg H, Block M, Madonia M *et al.* Treating major depression in primary care practice. Eight-month clinical outcomes. *Archives of General Psychiatry* 1996;53:913–19.

42 Corney R. Links between mental health professionals and general practices in England and Wales: the impact of GP fundholding. *British Journal of General Practice* 1996;46:221–4.

43 Sibbald B, Addington-Hall J, Brenneman D, Freeling P. Counsellors in English and Welsh general practices: their nature and distribution. *British Medical Journal* 1993;306:29–33.

44 Katon W, Schulberg H. Epidemiology of depression in primary care. *General Hospital Psychiatry* 1992;14:237–47.

45 Dowrick C, Gask L, Perry R, Dixon C, Usherwood T. Do general practitioners attitudes towards the management of depression predict their clinical behaviour? *Psychologcial Medicine* 2000;30:413–19.

46 Klinkman MS, Valenstein M. A general approach to psychiatric problems in the primary care setting. In: Knesper D, Riba M, Schwenk T, editors. *Primary Care Psychiatry*. Philadelphia: WB Saunders, 1997:3–8.

47 Ormel J, Koeter MWJ, van den Brink W, van den Willige G. Recognition, management and course of anxiety and depression in general practice. *Archives of General Psychiatry* 1991; 700–6.

48 Thompson C, Ostler K, Peveler RC. Dimensional perspective on the recognition of depressive symptoms in primary care. *British Journal of Psychiatry* 2001;179:317–23.

49 Gask L, Rogers A, Oliver D, Roland M. Qualitative study of patients' perceptions of the quality of care for depression in general practice. *British Journal of General Practice* 2000;53:278–83.

50 Khan N, Bower P, Rogers A. Guided self-help in primary care mental health Meta-synthesis of qualitative studies of patient experience. *British Journal of Psychiatry* 2007;191:206–11.

51 Kadam UT, Croft P, McLeod J. A qualitative study of patient's views on anxiety and depression. *British Journal of General Practice* 2001;51:375–80.

52 Burr J, Chapman T. Contextualising experiences of depression in women from South Asian communities: a discursive approach. *Sociology of Health and Illness* 2004;26:433–52.

53 Rogers A, May C, Oliver D. Experiencing depression, experiencing the depressed: the separate worlds of patients and doctors. *Journal of Mental Health* 2001;10:317–33.

54 Grime J, Pollock K. Information versus experience: a comparison of an information-leaflet on antidepressants with lay experience of treatment. *Patient Education and Counseling* 2004;54:361–8.

55 Maxwell M. Women's and doctors' accounts of their experiences of depression in primary care: the influence of social and moral reasoning on patients' and doctors' decisions. *Chronic Illness* 2005;1:61–71.

56 Knudsen P, Hansen E, Traulsen J. Changes in self-concept while using SSRI antidepressants. *Qualitative Health Research* 2002;12:932–44.

57 World Health Organization. *World Health Report 2001: Mental Health: New Understanding, New Hope*. Geneva: World Health Organization, 2001.

58 World Health Organization. *Constitution*. Geneva: World Health Organization, 1948.

59 Laine C, Davidoff F. Patient-centered medicine: a professional evolution. *Journal of the American Medical Association* 1996;275:152–6.

60 Department of Health. *Our Health, Our Care, Our Say: A New Direction for Community Services*. London: The Stationery Office, 2006.

2

Models of care for depression

Peter Bower and Simon Gilbody

Case study

Dr Stevens is a general practitioner in a busy inner city practice. She has a certain interest in mental health and spent some time in this specialty before coming into general practice. Most of her previous exposure to mental health had been in specialist mental health services where the majority of patients had problems such as schizophrenia.

Dr Stevens' managers have recently highlighted the need to improve the care for people with mental health problems, and have set aside funds to do this. She has taken it on herself to make this her responsibility. Many of her clinical colleagues already ask for her help and expertise and direct patients with mental health problems to her clinic.

Dr Stevens has set aside one session per week over the next six months and she is wondering what to do with this time. She could do more of what she already does by seeing more people with mental health problems. Alternatively, she knows that the practice will be rewarded if it institutes a screening programme for depression among those with long-term conditions. Another option she has considered is organizing an educational event on depression guidelines for herself and her partners. A useful leaflet offering a programme of seminars recently arrived in the post.

Dr Stevens has also wondered about using the money set aside for mental health to employ either a counsellor or clinical psychologist to work in the practice. Lastly, she wonders whether primary care is the best place to manage people with mental health problems, and she wonders about just asking her managers to use their resources to commission more care from the psychiatric or psychology services at the nearby mental health clinic. She lists this as an agenda item for the next meeting and wants to use research evidence to do the best thing for the practice population with the funds available.

Health services are complex, and making sense of that complexity is a challenge for patients, professionals and policy makers alike. Services are driven by a large

Depression in Primary Care: Evidence and Practice, ed. Simon Gilbody and Peter Bower. Published by Cambridge University Press. © Cambridge University Press 2011.

number of different factors: the characteristics of the patient population; the professional and other resources available in the locality; and aspects of local context such as history, culture and geography. Added to that are the changes associated with different quality improvement initiatives which may have been implemented, driven by either local enthusiasts or central government policy.

Given this complexity, the casual observer has a difficult job describing the various services which may be present in particular localities, and in identifying commonalities and differences between these services. This in turn makes it difficult to discover which services work best and which are less successful in meeting the policy goals outlined in Chapter 1. In these cases, conceptual models are often useful.

Conceptual models are abstract representations of complex areas, 'inventions of the human mind to place facts, events and theories in an orderly manner'.[1] These abstractions are designed to strip away some of the complexity in an area to focus on key issues of relevance. For example, it is possible to describe different types of dance in terms of a small number of categories (e.g. waltz, rumba). These categories are not supposed to capture everything of interest, and necessarily simplify the complex reality. But they are designed to highlight differences in content and process, to allow decision makers to concentrate on a smaller number of critical issues.

In the area of mental health, policy makers and service managers are faced with a huge number of disparate quality improvement interventions.[2] To reduce this complexity, we have described four 'models', which represent qualitatively different ways of quality improvement in depression. We do not claim that all the different ways that services can be configured are captured by these models. Instead, we think these models are useful ways of describing and thinking about quality improvement in depression.

Models of quality improvement in primary care mental health

Education and training model

In Chapter 1 we reviewed some of the research that suggests that many problems with delivery of care for depression in primary care relate to the knowledge, skills and attitudes of primary care professionals. The 'pathways to care' model (see Figure 1.1) highlights that firstly, one of the key pathways into treatment for depressed patients is through the recognition of their problems by the primary care professional. If this does not occur, access to care can be blocked at a very early stage.

Secondly, even if patients are recognized, deficiencies in the skills of primary care professionals can still lead to problems with quality of care. Although the effectiveness of antidepressant medication continues to be subject to debate,[3,4] medication remains a key part of the treatment of depression. For the purposes of this book, the issue is not the effectiveness of antidepressants per se, but the issue of how to best encourage professionals to prescribe them and patients to adhere to them. Evidence suggests that provision of antidepressant medication in primary care is often not in line with current best practice, with patients receiving inadequate doses of medication, for an inadequate duration.[5,6]

Similarly, although many patients appreciate the psychological support provided by primary care, there are concerns that such support is often not based on best evidence and representative of effective ways of intervening.[7] Finally, referral to specialist mental health professionals and other sources of support may not always be appropriate, with some patients referred who may not need specialist assistance, and others denied referral when they stand to benefit.

Training and education has been defined as 'the provision of essential knowledge and skills in the identification, prevention and care of mental disorders to primary health care personnel'.[8] Training may relate to diagnostic skills, or can focus on management, influencing the effective delivery of medication, or the use of communication skills and formal psychological therapy.[7] There are a number of methods for training and education, which differ in intensity, complexity and cost. Each will be described in some detail below.

At one level, training and education may involve large-scale public relations campaigns designed to change attitudes of professionals.[9] Such interventions are based on the assumption that problems in the delivery of quality mental healthcare in primary care are due (at least in part) to professional attitudes and beliefs about the prevalence, importance and treatability of depression, or issues such as stigma.[10,11] Some research has shown how such attitudes may relate to diagnostic behaviour.[12,13]

A good example of this model was the Defeat Depression campaign in the UK. This was run by the Royal College of Psychiatrists and the Royal College of General Practitioners, and was designed to enhance public awareness and provide professional education. This was achieved through a variety of means, and for professionals included 'an extensive program of general practice education … consensus conferences and statements, recognition and management guidelines, training videotapes, and other publications'.[9]

A second model of education and training is the dissemination of evidence-based guidelines.[14] Clinical guidelines are: [15]

systematically developed statements to assist practitioner and patient decisions about appropriate health care for specific clinical circumstances.

They may offer concise instructions on many aspects of healthcare practice, including screening, diagnosis, management and prevention. One of the earliest evidence-based guidelines produced in the USA was on depression.[16]

Guidelines can provide a lot of information and support for professionals. Box 2.1 includes some of the recommendations of the latest depression guidelines in the UK.[17] As can be seen, they include general statements about the way depressed patients should be treated, as well as more specific statements about preferred treatments (both in terms of what should be provided and what should not).

Box 2.1 Depression guidelines in the UK[17]

Information and consent

When working with people with depression and their families or carers:
- Build a trusting relationship and work in an open, engaging and non-judgemental manner
- Explore treatment options in an atmosphere of hope and optimism, explaining the different courses of depression and that recovery is possible.

Case identification

Be alert to possible depression (particularly in people with a past history of depression or a chronic physical health problem with associated functional impairment) and consider asking people who may have depression two questions, specifically:
- During the last month, have you often been bothered by feeling down, depressed or hopeless?
- During the last month, have you often been bothered by having little interest or pleasure in doing things?

Treatment options

For people with moderate or severe depression, provide a combination of antidepressant medication and a high-intensity psychological intervention.
The choice of intervention should be influenced by the:
- Duration of the episode of depression and the trajectory of symptoms
- Previous course of depression and response to treatment
- Likelihood of adherence to treatment and any potential adverse effects
- Person's treatment preference and priorities.

When an antidepressant is to be prescribed, it should usually be a selective serotonin uptake inhibitor in a generic form because these drugs are equally effective as other antidepressants and have a favourable risk–benefit ratio.

Although potentially powerful, the impact of guidelines in many areas of medicine has often been disappointing.[18] Guidelines are more effective with certain types of health problems (acute rather than chronic), when evidence is stronger, and when the guideline is compatible with existing values, skills and routine care processes.[19]

More intensive methods of training and education involve practice-based educational events.[20] The best example is the Hampshire Depression Project,[21] which sought to improve the recognition and management of depression through a realistic practice-based educational intervention involving four hours of teaching. The approaches used in that model are outlined in Box 2.2.

The most complex training and education programmes seek to make more fundamental changes to the attitudes and skills of primary care professionals, in order

> **Box 2.2** Training and education in the Hampshire Depression Project[20]
>
> ### Clinical practice guideline
>
> The guideline was based on a review of existing guidelines and included advice on practice organization, the roles of non-medical professionals, and a resource pack containing useful general and local information. The guideline was brief and flexible to allow modification and to promote ownership by primary care teams. The guideline recommended tricyclic antidepressants as first-line treatment but advised professionals to aim for a dose of 150 mg because of the lack of efficacy of low-dose tricyclics. Professionals were recommended to change to more tolerable medication if necessary.
>
> ### Education
>
> The education team included a primary care doctor, a practice nurse and a community mental health nurse. They were trained by a steering committee. Education was provided in two parts. Seminars were held at the beginning of the year for all members of the primary healthcare team. Each practice received four hours of seminars. Teaching was supplemented by videotapes to demonstrate interview and counselling skills, small-group discussion and role play. The educators remained available to the practices after training for additional assistance.

to teach advanced counselling and psychological therapy skills such as problem solving and cognitive-behavioural therapy. Such models are not easy to deliver through usual educational systems in primary care[22] and their complexity means that they are only likely to be of interest to a small number of primary care professionals. For this reason, we do not consider these programmes in detail, but interested readers are encouraged to examine relevant references.[7,23,24]

Consultation-liaison model

In some ways, the consultation-liaison model can be seen as a variant of the education and training model, in that it is fundamentally concerned with the same aim: improving the skills of primary care professionals. However, rather than providing discrete training courses and educational events that change attitudes and teach skills in the management of depressed patients in general, the consultation-liaison model uses mental health specialists to support primary care professionals in caring for *specific patients who are currently undergoing care*.[2,25] This is achieved by entering into an ongoing educational relationship with the primary care team, rather than providing one-off education and training.

The exact definition of consultation-liaison in primary care varies according to context. In the USA, the term is most commonly associated with psychiatric work in inpatient general hospital settings. Consultation-liaison has been defined broadly as 'any clinical or educational intervention provided for general medical personnel by mental health specialists, usually clinicians'.[26] Other definitions focus on the educational role, stating that consultation 'entails collaborative problem solving between a mental health specialist (the consultant) and one or more persons (the consultees) who are responsible for providing some form of psychological assistance to another (the client)'.[27]

In the UK, Gask and colleagues have used criteria that reflect the 'gate-keeping' role of the primary care professional in that healthcare system.[2] They see consultation-liaison models as being defined by the following core features:

- regular face-to-face contact between psychiatrist and primary healthcare team
- psychiatric referral only takes place after discussion at a face-to-face meeting
- some cases are managed by the primary healthcare team alone after discussion
- when referral does take place there is feedback to the primary healthcare team.

According to Katon and Gonzales,[28] consultation-liaison refers to processes at two distinct levels: liaison refers to educational work with the primary care professional, while consultation refers to direct patient contact. A further variant, the 'conjoint' model,[29,30] draws on both of these levels and involves joint consultation between the psychiatrist or other mental health specialist, patient and primary care professional.

Effective consultation-liaison may lead to more efficient use of specialist time, compared with specialists seeing patients directly. The model ensures that the primary care professional remains at the forefront of depression care. Consultation-liaison can improve care through a number of mechanisms. Discussions with a specialist around the care of the individual patient should improve the care of that patient. In addition, these discussions should develop the skills of the primary care professional more generally, meaning that the model may improve care for all those patients with depression, even those who are not the specific subject of liaison discussions with a specialist.

Collaborative care model

Recent years have seen the emergence of a new model of care called 'collaborative care'. This complex model has elements of both the educational and consultation-liaison model,[25] but in addition requires fundamental changes to the *system* of care. In Chapter 1, evidence was presented that depression is often a long-term condition, and the collaborative care model suggests that changes in the organization and delivery of services that have been introduced to improve the quality of care of long-term conditions such as diabetes are of equal relevance to depression.

The Chronic Care Model (www.improvingchroniccare.org) is the best known approach to the management of long-term conditions, and suggests that improvements in quality of care require a multilevel approach, intervening at the community, organization, professional and patient level. Care is designed to be proactive, and involves: following up patients; monitoring their outcomes; adjusting treatment plans when patients do not improve; and consulting with specialists when necessary. The model describes changes to the health system (to promote safe, high-quality care) and to the community (to mobilize resources to meet patient need), as well as four key changes to primary care practice.

- self-management support (providing information to enable the patient to care better for their problems)
- delivery system design (planning contacts in advance, involving a care team, each with clearly defined roles, close follow-up and attention to adherence)
- decision support (access to evidence-based practice guidelines and to professionals with relevant clinical expertise)
- clinical information systems (disease registers that can identify patients with specific needs, reminder systems to follow-up patients and monitor progress).

The full range of interventions in collaborative care models varies, but generally includes practitioner education and the provision of guidelines, screening and patient education,[31] augmented by changes in practice routines and developments in information technology.[32] Most importantly, collaborative care models are based on changes in roles. This includes changes to the roles of both primary care providers and specialists such as psychiatrists,[33] as well as the introduction of a new role – *the case manager*.

These different roles have been outlined in detail.[33] While the roles of the primary care provider and the specialist are similar to those in the training and consultation-liaison model, the introduction of the case manager is a major innovation, with the role involving assessment, behaviour change support, clinical management, ongoing follow-up and care coordination (Box 2.3).

The development of the case manager role is crucial to the collaborative care model, and a variety of methods of introducing this role have been described, including retraining existing staff[33] or the introduction of new mental health workers.[34]

Box 2.3 The role of the case manager in collaborative care[33]

Role of the case manager	Dimensions of the chronic care model
Assessment: regularly assess patient control of the illness, monitor success of the care plan, monitor improvement in condition	Self-management support Decision support
Behaviour change support: collaboratively develop a care plan that reflects treatment indications and patient preference	Self-management support
Clinical management: Provide intervention and adjust therapeutic regimen by protocol or discuss change with the primary care professional	Decision support Delivery system design
Ongoing follow-up: provide proactive follow-up, including support to maintain behaviour change	Clinical information systems Self-management support Delivery system design
Care coordination: coordinate care across the healthcare system and community resources. Facilitate transition by assisting patients to negotiate access	Health system and community resources

> **Box 2.4** Description of a collaborative care intervention in the IMPACT study of late-life depression[36]
>
> Patients receive an educational videotape and a booklet about late-life depression, and meet with a depression care manager (nurse or psychologist). The care manager conducts a detailed psychosocial history, reviews educational materials and discusses patient preferences for treatment.
>
> The care manager works with the patient and the primary care professional to deliver a treatment plan according to an algorithm, although patient choice is important. The algorithm suggests an initial choice of an antidepressant medication or a course of problem-solving treatment (a brief treatment for depression). New cases and cases needing adjustment to their management are discussed with a psychiatrist and a primary care physician. The care managers encourage patients to schedule pleasant life events and refer them to other professionals as required.
>
> Care managers follow patients for up to 12 months, monitoring treatment response with a standardized questionnaire and a web-based clinical information system. Patients who recover from depression develop a relapse prevention plan and then are followed up monthly. Patients who do not respond to initial treatment are discussed within the clinical team and further treatment delivered.

Collaborative care models are sometimes described as 'complex interventions', a term used to refer to interventions that 'comprise a number of separate elements that seem essential to the proper functioning of the intervention, although the *active ingredient* of the intervention that is effective is difficult to specify' [emphasis added].[35] An indication of the complexity of collaborative care is shown in Box 2.4, which outlines the IMPACT model of care for patients with late-life depression.[36]

Referral model

Although primary care clinicians always have overall clinical responsibility for their patients, in the referral model the management of the presenting problem is passed onto a mental health professional for the duration of the treatment.[37] This model is most frequently associated with the provision of psychological therapies in primary care. The use of such interventions has a relatively long history, dating back to innovators such as Balint, who identified the potential for psychological therapy in primary care, although he highlighted the role of the general practitioner rather than the mental health specialist.[38] In the UK the prevalence of depression and other disorders, combined with new flexibilities in funding, led to an explosion of the provision of such psychological therapies in primary care.[39] Such treatments were seen as providing a new referral option for hard-pressed primary care professionals, were associated with high levels of patient satisfaction and were assumed to lead to reductions in healthcare utilization, which meant that their costs might be offset by reductions in utilization in other parts of the healthcare system.[40]

There are many varieties of psychological therapy that have been provided in primary care, such as cognitive-behavioural therapy,[41] problem solving,[42] counselling[43] and interpersonal therapy.[44] There are major debates about their relative effectiveness and cost-effectiveness.[45–48] Unlike the previous models described in this chapter, there is little in the way of structured interaction between psychological therapist and primary care provider in this model. Indeed, one of the main drivers for the introduction of this model in the UK was the perception that bringing psychological therapists into primary care would free up the time of the primary care professional for other tasks. That is not to say that interactions do not occur. Professionals may interact in informal 'corridor consults', and the presence of a psychological therapist as part of the primary care team may have fundamental effects on practice attitudes, culture and organization. However, these are largely seen as beneficial side effects, rather than being seen as a key mechanism in this model.[49]

The relationships between models and policy goals

Clearly, these models differ in many important ways. For example, different professionals are involved in each model, and their interactions vary significantly. Specialists and primary care professionals may have only limited interaction in education and training models, whereas they are much more closely linked in the consultation-liaison model. New professionals are required in the collaborative care and referral models, while the collaborative care model may also require the introduction of organizational changes and new systems to support care. Models are also likely to differ in their costs and the challenges associated with their implementation.

However, for the purposes of the present book, one of the key dimensions along which these models differ relates to the importance of the primary care professional in the management of depression and the degree to which the model focuses on improving their skills and confidence (Figure 2.1). The primary care professional has the greatest involvement in the education and training model, because it is expected that they will deal with the bulk of mental health issues after training, with only a small proportion referred for specialist care. The involvement of the primary care professional is still significant in consultation-liaison, although the relative involvement of the specialist increases because they are involved in long-term relationships with primary care staff. In collaborative care models, the introduction of the case manager means that a significant proportion of the work that was originally the responsibility of the primary care professional is shifted to these new staff. Finally, in the referral model, the transfer of workload is greatest, and the responsibility of the primary care professional is potentially reduced the most.

This provides a link between quality improvement models, the 'pathways to care' model and policy goals such as access and equity. *Assuming equivalent*

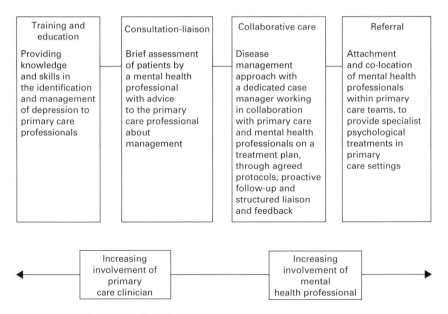

Figure 2.1 Models of mental healthcare in primary care.

effectiveness, those models that put greater focus on increasing the abilities of primary care professionals have the greatest potential impact on access and equity. This is because those models can most readily influence filter 2 and treatment at level 3 (see Figure 1.1), which can potentially influence the largest numbers of patients (i.e. all patients with common mental health problems presenting in primary care). In contrast, models that require significant specialist involvement at the level of the individual patient (such as collaborative care and referral) can only impact on the smaller proportion of patients who pass filter 3. If education and training can be shown to be effective, then the overall impact on the policy goals of access and equity will be maximized.

However, the key statement is 'assuming equivalent effectiveness'. In the context of evidence-based clinical practice and policy making, clinical and cost-effectiveness can no longer be assumed, but requires high-quality evidence from the most rigorous designs before particular models can be implemented.

Concluding comments

The following chapters outline the principles of evidence-based practice and methods for the synthesis of clinical and economic data. This will then set the stage for the standardized methods used to summarize current evidence concerning these models of depression care, which will explore their relative clinical and cost-effectiveness, and allow us to make policy recommendations for the future delivery of mental healthcare in primary care.

REFERENCES

1 Siegler M, Osmond H. *Models of Madness Models of Medicine*. New York: MacMillan, 1974.

2 Gask L, Sibbald B, Creed F. Evaluating models of working at the interface between mental health services and primary care. *British Journal of Psychiatry* 1997;170:6–11.

3 Moncrieff J, Wessely S, Hardy R. Meta-analysis of trials comparing antidepressants with active placebos. *British Journal of Psychiatry* 1998;172:227–31.

4 Kirsch I, Deacon B, Huedo-Medina T, Scoboria A, Moore T, Johnson B. Initial severity and antidepressant benefits: a meta-analysis of data submitted to the Food and Drug Administration. *PLOS Medicine* 2010;5:e45.

5 Katon W, Von Korff M, Lin E, Bush T, Ormel J. Adequacy and duration of antidepressant treatment in primary care. *Medical Care* 1992;30:67–6.

6 Katon W, Von Korff M, Lin E *et al.* Population-based care of depression: effective disease management strategies to decrease prevalence. *General Hospital Psychiatry* 1997;19:169–78.

7 King M, Davidson O, Taylor F, Haines A, Sharp D, Turner R. Effectiveness of teaching general practitioners skills in brief cognitive behaviour therapy to treat patients with depression: randomised controlled trial. *British Medical Journal* 2002;324:947–52.

8 World Health Organization. *ATLAS – Mental Health Resources in the World 2001*. Geneva: World Health Organization, 2001.

9 Priest R. A new initiative on depression. *British Journal of General Practice* 1991;41:487.

10 Cabana M, Rushton J, Rush J. Implementing practice guidelines for depression: applying a new framework to an old problem. *General Hospital Psychiatry* 2002;24:35–42.

11 Botega N, Mann A, Blizard R, Wilkinson G. General practitioners and depression – first use of the depression attitudes questionnaire. *International Journal of Methods in Psychiatric Research* 1992;2:169–80.

12 Marks J, Goldberg D, Hillier V. Determinants of the ability of general practitioners to detect psychiatric illness. *Psychological Medicine* 1979;9:337–53.

13 Dowrick C, Gask L, Perry R, Dixon C, Usherwood T. Do general practitioners' attitudes towards depression predict their clinical behaviour? *Psychological Medicine* 2000;30:413–19.

14 Cornwall P, Scott J. Which clinical practice guidelines for depression? An overview for busy practitioners. *British Journal of General Practice* 2000;50:908–11.

15 Field M, Lohr K. *Clinical Practice Guidelines: Directions for a New Program*. Washington, DC: National Academy Press, 1990.

16 Agency for Health Care Policy Research. *Depression in Primary Care*. Washington, DC: US Department of Health and Human Services, 1993.

17 National Institute for Health and Clinical Excellence. *Depression: the Treatment and Management of Depression in Adults (update)*. London: National Institute for Health and Clinical Excellence, 2009. Available at: www.nice.org.uk/nicemedia/pdf/Depression_Update_FULL_GUIDELINE.pdf

18 Grimshaw JM, Thomas RE, MacLennan G *et al.* Effectiveness and efficiency of guideline dissemination and implementation strategies. *Health Technology Assessment* 2004;8:1–72

19 Grol R, Grimshaw J. From best evidence to best practice: effective implementation of change in patients' care. *Lancet* 2003;362:1225–30.

20 Thompson C, Kinmonth A, Stevens L *et al*. Effects of a clinical practice guideline and practice-based education on detection and outcome of depression in primary care: Hampshire Depression Project randomised controlled trial. *Lancet* 2000;355:185–91.

21 Thompson C, Stevens L, Ostler K *et al*. The Hampshire Depression Project: a methodology for assessing the value of general practice education in depression. *International Journal of Methods in Psychiatric Research* 1996;6:S27–31.

22 Kendrick T. Why can't GPs follow guidelines on depression? *British Medical Journal* 2000;320:200–1.

23 Huibers M, Beurskens A, Bleijenberg G, Van Schayck C. The effectiveness of psychosocial interventions delivered by general practitioners. *Cochrane Database of Systematic Reviews* 2007;Issue 3:CD003494. DOI: 10.1002/14651858.CD003494.pub2.

24 Mynors-Wallis L, Gath D, Day A, Baker F. Randomised controlled trial of problem solving treatment, antidepressant medication, and combined treatment for major depression in primary care. *British Medical Journal* 2000;320:26–30.

25 Bower P, Gask L. The changing nature of consultation-liaison in primary care: bridging the gap between research and practice. *General Hospital Psychiatry* 2002;24:63–70.

26 Gonzales J, Norquist G. Mental health consultation-liaison interventions in primary care. In: J Miranda, A Hohmann, C Attkisson, D Larson, editors. *Mental Disorders in Primary Care*. San Francisco, CA: Jossey-Bass, 1994:347–73.

27 Medway F, Updyke J. Meta-analysis of consultation outcome studies. *American Journal of Community Psychology* 1985;13:489–505.

28 Katon W, Gonzales J. A review of randomised trials of psychiatric consultation-liaison studies in primary care. *Psychosomatics* 1994;35:268–79.

29 Dym B, Berman S. The primary health care team: family physician and family therapist in joint practice. *Family Systems Medicine* 1986;4:9–21.

30 Mitchell A. Psychiatrists in primary health care settings. *British Journal of Psychiatry* 1985;147:371–9.

31 Von Korff M, Goldberg D. Improving outcomes in depression. *British Medical Journal* 2001;323:948–9.

32 Wagner E, Austin B, Von Korff M. Organizing care for patients with chronic illness. *Milbank Quarterly* 1996;74:511–43.

33 Katon W, Von Korff M, Lin E, Simon G. Rethinking practitioner roles in chronic illness: the specialist, primary care physician and the practice nurse. *General Hospital Psychiatry* 2001;23:138–44.

34 Harkness E, Bower P, Gask L, Sibbald B. Improving primary care mental health: survey evaluation of an innovative workforce development in England. *Primary Care Mental Health* 2006;3:253–60.

35 Campbell M, Fitzpatrick R, Haines A *et al*. Framework for design and evaluation of complex interventions to improve health. *British Medical Journal* 2000;321:694–6.

36 Unützer J, Katon W, Callahan C *et al*, for the IMPACT investigators. Collaborative care management of late-life depression in the primary care setting: a randomized controlled trial. *Journal of the American Medical Association* 2003;288:2836–45.

37 Bower P. Primary care mental health workers: models of working and evidence of effectiveness. *British Journal of General Practice* 2002;52:926–33.

38 Balint M, Balint E. *Psychotherapeutic Techniques in Medicine*. London: Tavistock, 1961.

39 Sibbald B, Addington-Hall J, Brenneman D, Freeling P. Counsellors in English and Welsh general practices: their nature and distribution. *British Medical Journal* 1993;306:29–33.

40 Simpson S, Corney R, Fitzgerald P. Counselling provision, prescribing and referral rates in a general practice setting. *Primary Care Psychiatry* 2003;8:115–19.

41 Scott A, Freeman C. Edinburgh primary care depression study: treatment outcome, patient satisfaction, and cost after 16 weeks. *British Medical Journal* 1992;304:883–7.

42 Mynors-Wallis L, Davies I, Gray A, Barbour F, Gath D. A randomised controlled trial and cost analysis of problem-solving treatment for emotional disorders given by community nurses in primary care. *British Journal of Psychiatry* 1997;170:113–19.

43 Ward E, King M, Lloyd M *et al*. Randomised controlled trial of non-directive counselling, cognitive-behaviour therapy and usual GP care for patients with depression. I: Clinical effectiveness. *British Medical Journal* 2000;321:1383–8.

44 Schulberg H, Block M, Madonia M *et al*. Treating major depression in primary care practice: eight month clinical outcomes. *Archives of General Psychiatry* 1996;53:913–19.

45 Tarrier N. Commentary: Yes, cognitive-behaviour therapy may well be all you need. *British Medical Journal* 2002;324:291–2.

46 Bolsover N. Commentary: The 'evidence' is weaker than claimed. *British Medical Journal* 2002;324:294

47 Hinshelwood R. Commentary: Symptoms or relationships. *British Medical Journal* 2002;324:292–3.

48 Holmes J. All you need is cognitive-behaviour therapy. *British Medical Journal* 2002;324:288–90.

49 Harkness E, Bower P. On-site mental health workers delivering psychological therapy and psychosocial interventions to patients in primary care: effects on the professional practice of primary care providers. *Cochrane Database of Systematic Reviews* 2009;Issue 1:CD000532. DOI: 10.1002/14651858.CD000532.pub2.

3

Linking evidence to practice

Peter Bower and Simon Gilbody

Case study

Dr Stevens has a week to prepare for the forthcoming meeting about improving services for depression. She is keen that she uses the best evidence available to make an informed decision about service development and allocation of resources. She remembers a brief training event on 'skills for evidence-based practice', which she attended three years ago. In that session she learned about literature searching. She thinks an electronic search with some key words might help her find the relevant research. She types a number of key words into MEDLINE, including depression and primary care, and comes up with hundreds of 'hits', many of which refer to randomized controlled trials.

Dr Stevens tries to narrow this down a little by selecting only 'review' articles, and finds a list of papers – some of which are conventional review articles, and some of which call themselves 'systematic reviews', including 'Cochrane reviews'. She thinks this would be a good place to start and selects some that seem relevant. However, she reminds herself to do some background reading on systematic reviews.

Decision making is fundamental to healthcare. Faced with a patient in distress, any health professional will have to make a large number of decisions about the nature of the treatment that will be provided. Similarly, those who commission services or make decisions about health policy need to ensure that they invest in effective services, and get the greatest return on their investment in terms of health and well-being. Clearly, such decisions have major implications, and there is interest in improving the way those decisions are made, by linking decision making more clearly to scientific evidence. This has often been identified with a movement called 'evidence-based medicine' or 'evidence-based practice'.

As noted in Chapter 1, evidence-based practice was defined by one of its originators as 'the conscientious, explicit, and judicious use of current best evidence in making decisions about the care of individual patients'.[1] In some ways, this

Depression in Primary Care: Evidence and Practice, ed. Simon Gilbody and Peter Bower. Published by Cambridge University Press. © Cambridge University Press 2011.

statement is uncontroversial, because few would argue that 'evidence' about the effectiveness of treatments should guide decision-making. However, initial debates have centred on the types of evidence that should inform decision making.[2] These debates have been followed by additional arguments about the importance placed on evidence about what treatments are 'effective' (i.e. the *clinical effectiveness* of treatments in reducing symptoms and improving quality of life) and how 'effective' interventions are prioritized within constrained healthcare budgets (i.e. the *cost-effectiveness* of interventions, in terms of achieving clinical effectiveness at a reasonable and sustainable cost).[3] Knowledge of clinical effectiveness is necessary but not sufficient for decisions about healthcare delivery, since evidence about clinical effectiveness gives little information on the amount of resources required to generate particular outcomes.

The key design that has emerged to judge clinical effectiveness is the randomized controlled trial, and the most rigorous means of judging cost effectiveness is the use of economic analyses within or alongside randomized controlled trials.[4]

Randomized controlled trials in evidence-based practice

A randomized controlled trial is an example of an *experiment*, where the researcher actively manipulates some parameters (called *independent variables*) and then examines the effect of this manipulation on other parameters (called *dependent variables*). Experiments are designed to remove the effect of *confounders*.

Confounders are variables that can confuse the issue of what is causing what. For example, if we provide a treatment to depressed patients and measure their outcome before and after treatment, we cannot be sure that the treatment is responsible for any change we observe. Depression is related to many factors other than treatment, such as the patient's pre-existing personality or changes in their life situation. These other influences are known as *confounders* and they make it unclear whether any one factor (such as treatment) can be held responsible for any changes in outcomes.[5,6]

Experiments are designed to improve our confidence that a relationship between an independent and dependent variable is 'causal', i.e. the treatment causes outcomes and can be said to 'work'. This confidence about causal relationships is described as *internal validity*.[7] Randomized trials are designed to provide the best protection against threats to internal validity. This is done through *comparison* (largely through the use of control groups, whose outcome can be compared with a treatment group); and *randomization* (allocating patients to treatments on the basis of chance).

Comparison in randomized controlled trials

Comparison means that different groups of patients receive different levels or types of treatment. A common type of randomized controlled trial is the 'no treatment' comparison, where one group receives a treatment and another group receives none. The exact meaning of 'no treatment' can vary. It may mean no treatment at all in certain contexts. Often, it means 'usual care' or 'treatment as usual', which means that patients receive the care that they would usually have access to and which will not generally include the treatment under test. A final common form of 'no treatment' group is a waiting list control, where some patients get immediate access to a treatment, and others are randomly allocated to a waiting list, to receive the treatment after a delay. The latter have their outcome measured at the end of the waiting list period, prior to receiving the treatment. There are important differences between these types of 'no treatment control', but they are sometimes treated as broadly comparable.

Alternatively, in other study designs patients may be allocated to two treatments (often called an 'active comparison' study). This may involve patients being given different amounts of the same treatment (e.g. comparing a brief and a more intensive psychological therapy, or a group or individual therapy) or two entirely different treatments (e.g. psychological therapy versus medication). It is possible for trials to have different numbers of treatment and comparison arms. For example, a study may have three 'active comparisons' (e.g. psychological therapy versus two different types of medication) or two 'active comparisons' and a 'no treatment' control (e.g. psychological therapy versus antidepressants versus usual care).

Randomization and selection bias

Randomization is crucial. Control and other comparison groups provide protection against confounders with one critical proviso: 'all other things being equal'. If the patients making up the treatment and control groups differ significantly in important characteristics (for example, the severity of their disorders) at the start of the experiment, then our conclusions will be suspect because these differences could very well account for any observed differences in outcome. This threat to the comparability of the groups at baseline is called *selection bias*.[7,8]

The answer is to allocate patients to treatment or control groups at random. With sufficient numbers of patients, this should ensure that there are no systematic differences on any variable between the groups. This means that any differences in outcome cannot be related to any pre-existing differences between the groups, because the groups are essentially equal. Randomization also ensures that the groups will be equal on *all* variables, both those that have been measured and those that are unmeasured.

Reporting the use of randomization is not enough to avoid selection bias. It is necessary that randomization is done correctly. This means that the decision about whether a patient is eligible to participate in a trial is separate from knowledge of the next allocation in the random sequence (and thus the decision about which treatment they will receive). For example, when entering a patient in a trial, it is important that the patient's eligibility is not altered because the clinician knows that the next treatment allocation is one that is viewed as unfavourable (for example, to a no-treatment control group). Bias is less likely where allocation is adequately *concealed*. The best way to do this is by separating people judging who is eligible for the trial from those who keep the random sequence, through so-called central randomization. In this system, the person judging eligibility makes that judgement and then receives the allocation via the telephone or Internet. Using this method, there is no way that the person can determine the next allocation in the sequence, which means that prior knowledge of the allocation cannot influence judgements of eligibility. The various issues concerning the process of randomization and the systems required to achieve high quality allocation have been discussed in detail in the literature.[9,10,11]

Power and sample size

The core function of a randomized controlled trial is to test whether the outcomes of patients in the randomized groups are different. The most common way of doing this is through a test of the statistical significance of the difference in the outcomes of those groups. Readers are urged to consult one of the many statistical textbooks available for a detailed explanation, but the basic idea is that tests of statistical significance explore whether the differences found between treatment and control groups (e.g. in the proportion of patients who recover from depression) are greater than that expected by chance. If the test suggests those differences are greater than those expected by chance, then the differences must be due to something other than chance. In a well-conducted randomized experiment, the *only* difference between the groups is the treatment, and thus we can confidently assume that the treatment is the causal factor.

A key concept that needs to be understood is *power*. One problem with statistical significance testing is that it is possible that a significant difference exists, but that we have been unable to detect it with our test. This is most likely to occur when we have insufficient patients in our trial (the number of patients is often called the *sample size*), and the test is said to lack power. In trials, it is important that we design the study and recruit sufficient patients to provide us with sufficient power. How do we decide what is sufficient? There is a procedure that must be followed called a *sample size calculation*. Again, the details can be found in statistical textbooks, but essentially the calculation involves determining the sort of difference that we want to detect, setting a level of power, and then using a formula to determine how many patients we would need in the study.

To give an example, we might say that we wish to detect whether our new medication treatment improves the proportion of patients recovering from depression. If we know from previous research that the recovery rate in current treatment is 40%, we might suggest that we are interested in an increase in the rate of recovery to 50%. Power (the probability we will detect a difference of this size when it actually exists) is usually set to 80% or 90%. Using those data (plus some other standard parameters), we can determine how many patients we need to achieve that level of power. If the new medication improves recovery rates by much more (say 20%) we will definitely have power to detect that. If the actual difference between treatments is smaller (say 5%), we may fail to detect it. However, we have already determined that we are not interested in such a difference, so our lack of power is less important.

Working out what sort of differences between treatment and control group are of interest is a complex issue,[12] which needs to take into account scientific and logistical issues, as well as value judgements about the worth of treatments. A treatment that shows greater differences in outcome between treatment and control group than would be expected by chance is said to demonstrate 'statistical significance'. Where there is agreement that the differences are worthwhile, a treatment is said to show differences of 'clinical significance'. If a trial is very small, it may not have adequate statistical power to detect clinically significant differences, while a very large trial may be able to detect differences between treatments that are statistically significant but that are so small as to be clinically meaningless.[13,14]

Many trials in the literature lack power, either because they have not done a sample size calculation, or because they have not been able to recruit all the patients they needed.[15,16] One of the functions of systematic reviews and meta-analysis is to overcome these limitations by pooling the results of several studies to increase power.

Cluster trials

Most trials randomize individual patients, but this is not always the case. Some interventions (such as education and training, consultation-liaison and some models of collaborative care) attempt to change the behaviour of professionals, which means that the changes will potentially benefit all patients who consult that professional. If individual patients are randomized to a collaborative care intervention or a control, and patients in the control group then attend a professional who has been trained in collaborative care, this can lead to *contamination*. This is where the effects of an intervention influence both randomized groups, potentially masking the effect of the intervention because it is inadvertently present in both groups. In those cases, a cluster randomized trial can be used, which involves randomizing professionals or even organizations, so that it is much easier to keep the intervention separate from the control groups. There are methodological,[17,18] statistical[19,20] and ethical issues[21,22] that must be taken into account in making sense of cluster trials, but the basic logic is the same as a patient randomized study.

Other issues in the quality of randomized controlled trials

There are many other issues to consider in the design, analysis and interpretation of randomized controlled trials.[9] Two key issues are concerned with the behaviour of patients in a trial after randomization, in relation to (a) the treatment under test, and (b) the assessments needed to assess the effects of those treatments (so-called outcome assessments).

In any trial, some patients do not receive their treatment as planned. Although it is possible to exclude such patients from the analysis (in what is called a *completer* or *on-treatment* analysis), such an approach can lead to selection bias, because the comparability between groups that randomization provides is lost if some patients are removed in a systematic fashion. The preferred approach is to include all patients once randomized, irrespective of whether they attended for or received treatment. This is called an *intention to treat analysis* and it preserves the benefits of randomization.[23]

Patients who take part in trials often drop out from their outcome assessments for various reasons, and do not provide data. This is described as *loss to follow-up* or *attrition bias*.[24] This bias can occur if many patients drop out and fail to provide outcome assessments, and is especially problematic if loss to follow-up is related to their outcome (i.e. dissatisfied patients may be more likely to leave the trial) or is unbalanced between arms (so that more patients drop out of one group or the other). Therefore, it is important to keep as many patients in the trial as possible, to ensure that the comparability between the groups that is created through randomization is maintained.

It is generally accepted that many treatments may work in part because of the expectation of recovery brought about by the offer of treatment.[25] For example, if patients are allocated to treatment or no treatment conditions, they will develop specific expectations about their outcome based on their allocation. In trials of medication, it is possible to overcome this problem by *blinding* patients and their clinicians to the treatment group to which they have been allocated, e.g. by using tablets that have identical characteristics, so that patients and professionals are unaware of which treatment they have received.[26] However, in the sorts of interventions discussed in this book, this is very difficult to achieve, because receiving an active intervention such as collaborative care cannot be easily disguised.

One form of blinding that is more relevant is observer blinding. When a researcher judges patient outcome at the end of the trial, it is important that they are not aware of which treatment the patient has received, otherwise this may cause bias in their assessments (so-called *detection bias*). Observer blinding can be difficult to achieve in practice, as patients will often inadvertently discuss their treatment during outcome assessments. In addition, many outcome assessments in mental health are completed by the patients (so-called self-report measures) where blinding is less relevant.

The *Cochrane Handbook* provides further detail about common forms of bias in randomized controlled trials (see www.cochrane-handbook.org).

Explanatory and pragmatic trials

Much of the focus within evidence-based practice is on the internal validity of studies, i.e. the degree to which the comparison of treatment and control can be considered unbiased, through techniques such as randomization, concealment of allocation, and low levels of attrition. There has been less focus on the issue of *external validity*, defined as the confidence with which a researcher can expect relationships found in the context of one particular experiment to *generalize* to other contexts. For example, will the relationships hold true in different settings, with different therapists, patients, and at different times?[27]

Although studies high on internal and external validity are the ideal, in practice there is often conflict between the two types of validity, such that there is a trade-off between the scientific rigour of a study and its external validity. This is because the conditions that optimize the former (i.e. randomization, comparison and control) are so rarely features of real-world settings to which the results are to be generalized.[7,28,29] A number of factors have been described that might potentially limit the external validity of trials,[30] including: levels of therapist training; the quality and format of treatments provided; the use of combination treatments; multiple roles for the therapist; homogeneity of patients entered into the trial; and the type of control group used.

Depending on the way in which trials deal with such threats to external validity, they can be described as *explanatory* or *pragmatic* in nature.[31,32] Explanatory trials require high levels of control over variables to provide rigorous demonstrations of the causal link between treatment and outcome. Interventions are clearly specified, the effects of expectations are controlled through use of placebos, and the types of patient entering the trial are defined by a rigid protocol. Such trials prioritize internal validity to answer basic scientific questions.

In contrast, pragmatic trials seek to balance internal and external validity to provide results that are more generalizable to routine settings than the specialized conditions usually found in explanatory trials. Treatments are provided flexibly, in that the exact nature of the treatment is left to the judgement of the clinician, and there is variation in quality and process of care as would be found in routine settings. Expectancies and other effects that can affect outcome are not usually controlled through placebos and blinding: if one treatment is viewed more favourably by patients, then such views are considered part of normal practice and a component of the treatment itself. Furthermore, it is not necessary that all patients attend for treatment, since failure to attend is a common aspect of clinical work, and intention-to-treat analyses (see above) are the norm. Whereas an explanatory design tries to provide the best test that a specific treatment is responsible for change, a pragmatic trial is concerned with the additional value associated with a broad treatment policy (i.e. offering patients access to a collaborative care intervention, for example). Although pragmatic trials do not seek to *control* key variables, it is important that they *report* the values that those variables took (e.g. the training and experience of the therapists) so that the conditions of the trial (and their relationship to routine practice) can be clearly judged. Issues in reporting are considered in more detail below.

Reporting of trials

Making sense of trials can be complex, and this is made even more difficult if the trial is reported poorly. To improve the reporting of trials, a standard has been set through the CONSORT Statement. CONSORT stands for CONsolidated Standards of Reporting Trials, and the statement is described as:

an evidence-based, minimum set of recommendations for reporting RCTs [randomized controlled trials]. It offers a standard way for authors to prepare reports of trial findings, facilitating their complete and transparent reporting, and aiding their critical appraisal and interpretation. (www.consort-statement.org)

The two core aspects of CONSORT are a 22-item checklist to assist in trial reporting, and a diagram which is designed to provide a very clear description of patient flow through a trial, including issues relating to attrition, adherence and intention-to-treat analyses. An example checklist item is the requirement that trials report methods used to implement the random allocation sequence (e.g. central telephone randomization), clarifying whether allocation was concealed until interventions were assigned.

An example CONSORT diagram is show in Figure 3.1, which divides the flow of patients in a trial into four stages: enrolment; allocation; follow-up; and analysis. Not all CONSORT diagrams will look the same (i.e. the diagram will differ for a three-arm trial, a trial with more than one follow-up, and a cluster trial), and some modification will be necessary for each, but the core of the diagram should be similar.

As well as a CONSORT diagram, another important part of the reporting of trials is the 'table of baseline characteristics'. One obvious check on the success of randomization is to actually compare the initial or 'baseline' characteristics of the randomized groups. Most published studies provide this sort of information in a table that places data about the treatment and control groups side by side. Visual inspection of the table can help to determine whether any bias has crept in. Sometimes, such differences indicate that there have been problems with the process of randomization or concealment of allocation. Even when studies are randomized properly, if there are relatively few patients, it is possible that selection bias can still occur. Some trials test the 'statistical significance' of these differences. If the differences are not 'statistically significant', some authors claim that this means that no bias is present. However, this procedure is flawed, because very small studies lack power. Small trials are therefore most likely to claim that there are no differences between groups, and most likely to be vulnerable to such differences.

It is possible to use statistical controls to ameliorate the effects of differences between groups at baseline, but this process is limited to those variables that have been measured – one of the great benefits of randomization is that it should provide comparability for all variables, measured or otherwise. Current guidance suggests that the choice of such controls should be based more on theoretical considerations than examining differences at baseline.[33] Nevertheless, a table of baseline characteristics is always a useful part of the presentation of a trial.

Systematic reviews in evidence-based practice

Although a well-conducted randomized controlled trial provides the best test of clinical and cost-effectiveness, each trial provides only a single test. A key scientific principle is the need for replication, as each additional study increases the accuracy of our knowledge and the confidence that particular results were not due to chance or the specific context in which a trial was done.

A key type of scientific publication is the review, which brings together studies on a topic. The popularity of review articles is a recognition that practitioners and policy makers need digestible forms of evidence that summarize research in an efficient and replicable manner.[34] Finding and appraising all the research evidence in

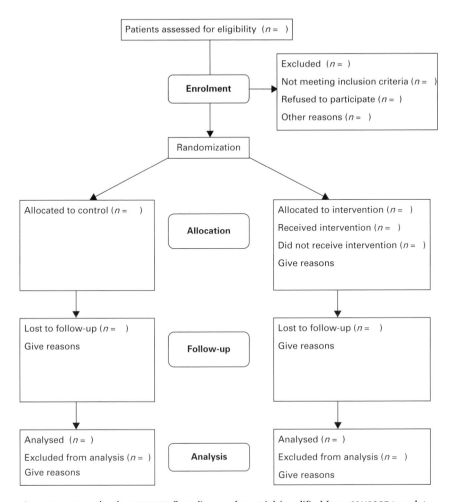

Figure 3.1 Example of a CONSORT flow diagram for a trial (modified from CONSORT template at www.consort-statement.org).

an area is a daunting task. Consequently, review articles are always popular among those who conduct and use research. However, it has been suggested that many review articles are open to bias and lack transparency.[35] For example, individual primary research studies often use different methods and differ in their rigour. How are we to make sense of such evidence? Another problem is that authors of reviews can be either consciously or unconsciously selective in the research they include. To avoid these sources of bias requires a specific type of review: the systematic review.

Systematic reviews seek to draw together individual primary research studies in order to provide an overview that is more comprehensive, accurate and generalizable than the results of individual studies. The aim of systematic reviews is to ensure that all potential sources of bias are made explicit and, where possible, minimized. This is achieved by a number of methods.

Explicit research question

Firstly, a systematic review starts with an explicit research question. These questions are often formulated according to the PICO algorithm (Population, Intervention, Comparison, Outcome). For example, the question 'Is psychotherapy worthwhile?' is a question of interest to professionals, managers, patients and taxpayers, but it is not a *scientific* question. The PICO approach enables us to turn such a general query into a specific question that can be effectively answered using scientific methods. In this case, an alternative question is: 'In patients with major depression (Population), is cognitive-behavioural therapy (Intervention) more effective than antidepressant medication (Comparison) in reducing depressive symptoms and avoiding relapse (Outcome)?'

Systematic reviews also make explicit the types of evidence needed to answer the question. This is often restricted to randomized controlled trials, but can include almost any study design in principle.

Comprehensive searches for studies

A core weaknesses of many reviews is that they are restricted to the literature that happens to be known to the individual reviewer. To avoid bias, systematic reviews need to have a comprehensive overview of the evidence, rather than reviewing only a selected part that happens to be available. The rise of evidence-based practice has led to advances in the technology of searching for literature, harnessing the power of bibliographic databases such as MEDLINE, EMBASE and PsycInfo.[36] There is increasing knowledge about which databases need to be searched, how to search them and the different biases that emerge from reliance on databases, such as *publication bias* (that is, the tendency for published studies to be atypical, especially in terms of a higher likelihood of reporting positive results).[37]

Quality appraisal

Systematic reviews seek to sort good-quality evidence from biased and misleading evidence through quality appraisal. A number of aspects of study design (such as randomization and concealment of allocation) have been shown to introduce bias, and appraisal of the quality of methods of randomisation and concealment of allocation remain the cornerstone of quality assessment within systematic reviews of randomized controlled trials. Other aspects of study design include the handling of attrition[23] and ensuring unbiased assessment of outcome.[26] In a systematic review, quality issues such as these are appraised using standardized checklists used by multiple independent raters, to assess the overall quality of the evidence in a rigorous and replicable manner, and to examine whether there is a consistent relationship between the quality of studies and their eventual outcomes. If such a relationship exists, then including studies of poor quality may systematically bias the results of the review. A significant debate exists about how best to measure quality.[38]

Synthesis

Systematic reviews synthesize primary research in order to highlight consistencies and differences between individual studies, and to provide a more accurate estimate of the relationships between treatments and their effects. Sometimes this synthesis is narrative. In this case, studies are described in terms of their design and results, and important areas of consistency and disagreement between individual studies are explored. The reviewer will attempt to summarize the totality of the evidence from these descriptions and the patterns that emerge. Narrative synthesis is most effective when there are a small number of studies in a review. As the number of studies increases, describing the literature in such a narrative fashion becomes more difficult because the level of detail can overwhelm even the most dedicated reader.

The most common mathematical tool used for quantitative synthesis of multiple studies is meta-analysis.[39,40] Although the terms systematic review and meta-analysis are sometimes used interchangeably, they are not identical, since a meta-analysis is not necessary for a systematic review, nor is meta-analysis sufficient to make a review systematic. In meta-analysis, primary studies deemed sufficiently similar in terms of setting, population, intervention and outcome are statistically summarized to get an overall estimate of effectiveness.

There are two stages to a meta-analysis. Firstly, the results of individual studies are calculated using a common method, to derive an estimate of the effectiveness of each treatment (the *effect size*). This can be in terms of the proportions of patients showing a particular outcome (if the outcome is *dichotomous* with only two states, such as being 'recovered' or 'not recovered' after treatment). Alternatively, this may involve the mean (average) score on a particular outcome measure (if the outcome is *continuous*, such as the score on a scale that measures the number and severity of symptoms of depression). For each trial, the difference in proportions or differences in mean scores between the comparison groups (e.g. between treatment and control) is calculated and translated to a common scale (Box 3.1).

The second stage involves *pooling* the results from individual trials. Although the technical aspects of pooling are beyond the scope of this book, it essentially involves calculating a weighted average of the individual study results, with larger studies given more prominence. This pooled analysis yields an average estimate of effectiveness for a particular intervention across a number of randomized controlled trials. The results of meta-analyses are most readily presented using a specific form of graph (a forest plot). An example of a forest plot from a published study[46] is given in Figure 3.2, with the important features noted.

Estimates of effectiveness (such as effect sizes) should be presented with a measure of the *precision* of that estimate, normally in terms of a 95% confidence interval. Confidence intervals are important. Even if studies are well designed and largely free from bias, the estimate of effectiveness is always likely to differ from the 'true' value because of the effect of random variation. The 95% confidence interval can be interpreted as the range of scores within which the 'true' measure of effectiveness is very likely to lie. All other things being equal, if studies include

Box 3.1 Calculation of an effect size

A randomized controlled trial assesses the effect of a treatment by comparing the outcomes in the treatment and control groups. Many measures of depression are continuous, providing a score that varies between 0 (where patients have no symptoms) up to a maximum based on the number and severity of symptoms a patient reports. For example, the Beck Depression Inventory has a score that ranges from 0 to 63.[41]

Comparing the mean scores of patients in the treatment and control groups gives a good indication of the impact of the treatment. For example, if patients in the treatment group have a mean score at the end of the study of 15, and the controls have a mean of 20, the *mean difference* is 5 points (i.e. treatment leads to a reduction in depression of 5 points on average). One difficulty is that it takes an expert to know whether a difference of 5 points is clinically important or trivial. A second problem is that studies often use different measures. Knowing that a treatment causes a mean reduction in depression of 5 points when depression has been measured on two completely different scales makes comparison impossible.

Effect sizes overcome these difficulties by *standardizing*. Essentially, this involves dividing the mean difference from each trial by a measure of the underlying variability of the scores on that outcome (the *standard deviation*). If scores are generally very variable, then a large mean difference would be required to demonstrate that treatment was better than control. If scores do not vary a lot, then a small mean difference may still represent an important effect of treatment. The mean difference divided by a measure of variability is often described as an *effect size*.

Standardizing in this way means that the difference between treatment and control groups can be described in terms of the same unit (i.e. units of standard deviation). So if one randomized controlled trial finds a mean difference of 5 points, and the standard deviation is 10, then the effect size is 0.5 (and the difference between depression scores of the treatment and control group is half a standard deviation). A second trial using a different measure might report a larger mean difference of 15, but if the standard deviation of scores in that trial is 25, then the effect size is actually only slightly increased (15/25 = 0.6) even though the mean difference is much larger.

A convention has emerged to judge the magnitude of effect sizes calculated in this way. An effect size of around 0.2 is often described as 'small', an effect size of 0.5 as 'medium' and an effect size of 0.8 as 'large'.[42] These are convenient labels with some validity,[12,43] and decision makers need to be careful in their interpretation, but they provide a useful rule of thumb to assess the effect of interventions in the context of the wider literature. Effect sizes are often reported as negative numbers in depression trials, because the effect of treatment is to reduce the number and severity of symptoms compared with patients who received no treatment. Further details on a variety of effect size calculations (including the appropriate calculations to use when outcome data are in dichotomous categories (e.g. 'depressed'/'not depressed') are available.[39,44,45]

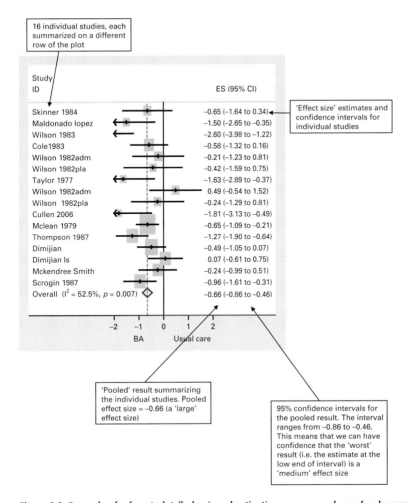

16 individual studies, each summarized on a different row of the plot

Study ID		ES (95% CI)
Skinner 1984		−0.65 (−1.64 to 0.34)
Maldonado lopez		−1.50 (−2.65 to −0.35)
Wilson 1983		−2.60 (−3.98 to −1.22)
Cole1983		−0.58 (−1.32 to 0.16)
Wilson 1982adm		−0.21 (−1.23 to 0.81)
Wilson 1982pla		−0.42 (−1.59 to 0.75)
Taylor 1977		−1.63 (−2.89 to −0.37)
Wilson 1982adm		0.49 (−0.54 to 1.52)
Wilson 1982pla		−0.24 (−1.29 to 0.81)
Cullen 2006		−1.81 (−3.13 to −0.49)
Mclean 1979		−0.65 (−1.09 to −0.21)
Thompson 1987		−1.27 (−1.90 to −0.64)
Dimijian		−0.49 (−1.05 to 0.07)
Dimijian Is		0.07 (−0.61 to 0.75)
Mckendree Smith		−0.24 (−0.99 to 0.51)
Scrogin 1987		−0.96 (−1.61 to −0.31)
Overall (I^2 = 52.5%, p = 0.007)		−0.66 (−0.86 to −0.46)

−2 −1 0 1 2
BA Usual care

'Effect size' estimates and confidence intervals for individual studies

'Pooled' result summarizing the individual studies. Pooled effect size = −0.66 (a 'large' effect size)

95% confidence intervals for the pooled result. The interval ranges from −0.86 to −0.46. This means that we can have confidence that the 'worst' result (i.e. the estimate at the low end of interval) is a 'medium' effect size

Figure 3.2 **Example of a forest plot (behavioural activation versus usual care for depression).**[41]

more patients, then precision will increase and the confidence intervals will narrow. *Precision* is different to *bias*. Bias is the degree to which our estimates deviate systematically from the truth, whereas precision is the degree of uncertainty in our knowledge. We can be precisely wrong (where we have a large, but poorly conducted, trial), or correct but imprecise (with a small but rigorous study), so it is important to distinguish these issues.

Confidence intervals are critical for interpretation. For example, a review may report an estimate of effect size of 0.5 (a 'medium' effect) and 95% confidence intervals of 0.4 to 0.6. In this case, we can be fairly sure that the 'true' effect is of 'medium' magnitude (see Box 3.1), because the 95% confidence intervals are quite close to the 0.5 value. If the review reported the same estimate of effect size of 0.5, but 95% confidence intervals of 0.2 to 0.8, the estimate is less precise, and we are less confident in our decision making. This is because it is eminently possible that the effect is actually 'large' or 'small' in magnitude, because the 95% confidence intervals include those values. In making decisions, we need to consider whether our decision would be the same if the effect size was actually at either end of the confidence interval. If it is not, we can have less confidence that we are making the right decision: more evidence may be needed.

Confidence intervals are also related to issues of statistical significance. If a study uses a continuous measure of outcome (e.g. a score on a depression scale measuring number and intensity of symptoms) and the confidence intervals around an effect size include 0 (i.e. the interval straddles both positive and negative effect sizes), then by definition the treatment does not show a statistically significant effect on outcome. If the confidence intervals do not include 0, the treatment has shown a statistically significant effect on outcome. This is why reporting of confidence intervals is much preferred to statements about statistical significance alone, as confidence intervals include all the information provided by the latter, but provide much more information as well.

Another important issue in meta-analysis is *heterogeneity*. The results of individual studies in a meta-analysis will always vary, even if the studies are essentially identical: this is simply the result of the play of chance.[47] However, on many occasions the variation is greater than would be expected by chance. This is described as *statistical heterogeneity*, and may be due to variability in the types of patients included in the studies, the different interventions under test or variation in the quality of the studies. High levels of heterogeneity suggest to some that it is inappropriate to pool studies in a meta-analysis, because the pooled estimate will give a misleading impression of an 'average' effect from studies that differ markedly in their individual effects. However, heterogeneity can also be explored using a variety of methods, and sometimes reasons for heterogeneity can be discovered that have important scientific, clinical and policy implications. For example, the effects of studies may be different in different contexts, or in different patient populations, or interventions including certain key 'ingredients' may be particularly effective. Heterogeneity can be assessed using a variety of methods, but a common index is the I^2 value, which gives an estimate of the amount of variation beyond that expected by chance. A rule of thumb is that an I^2 value of 25% is 'low', 50% is 'moderate' and 75% is 'high'.[48]

Estimates of heterogeneity are important in determining the exact statistical techniques to use in pooling studies. Although the issues are beyond the scope of the book, there are two main techniques for pooling called fixed-effect and random-effects,[39] that make different statistical assumptions and 'weight' the studies differently when they are pooled. Generally, fixed-effect models provide more precision (narrower confidence intervals), but when heterogeneity is high, random-effects models are generally more appropriate.

Quality assessment of systematic reviews

As noted above, quality assessment is a key part of a systematic review, but quality criteria can also be applied to reviews. For example, reviews can be assessed in

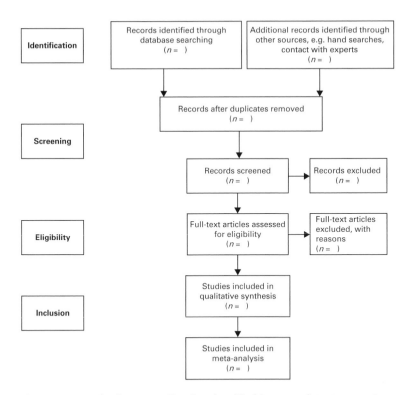

Figure 3.3 Example of a PRISMA flowchart (modified from template at www.prisma-statement.org/statement.htm).

terms of the degree to which the search was comprehensive, and whether rigorous procedures were used to assess the eligibility of studies and their quality (for example, use of two independent raters).

One key issue relates to the reporting of a systematic review. Like trials and the CONSORT statement, guidelines have been developed to improve the reporting of systematic reviews. These used to be known as QUOROM (*QU*ality *Of R*eporting *Of M*eta-analyses) but the latest version is called PRISMA (*P*referred *R*eporting *I*tems for *S*ystematic reviews and *M*eta-*A*nalyses, www.prisma-statement.org). The PRISMA guidelines state the sort of information that should be provided so that a reader can judge whether a review has been done well. Like CONSORT, PRISMA has a checklist of 27 items for reporting. For example, in reporting a search, PRISMA states that a report of a review should 'describe all information sources (e.g., databases with dates of coverage, contact with study authors to identify additional studies) in the search and date last searched'. Like CONSORT, PRISMA also has a flowchart that provides detail about four key stages in the review process: identification, screening, eligibility and inclusion (Figure 3.3). As with CONSORT, the exact nature of the flow diagram may vary, but the common core should remain the same.

Sources of systematic reviews

Given the prominence of systematic reviews, readers should be aware of two import-ant sources of these types of publication: the Cochrane Collaboration (and its publi-cation the *Cochrane Library*) and the Database of Abstracts of Reviews of Effects.

The Cochrane Collaboration is an international collaborative research effort to summarize all randomized trials across health and social care (see www.cochrane. org). Within this collaboration, a number of groups focused on mental health have formed. The Cochrane Depression Anxiety and Neurosis Group produces reviews in the area of depression. Cochrane reviews are produced using methods laid down by international methodological experts in the Collaboration (detailed in the *Cochrane Handbook*).[49] A fully searchable, freely accessible database of Cochrane reviews is available (www.thecochranelibrary.com).

The Database of Abstracts of Reviews of Effects is a database that records all known systematic reviews and is produced and maintained by the Centre for Reviews and Dissemination at the University of York (funded by the UK Department of Health). Importantly, researchers at this centre read all system-atic reviews that are produced and create a parallel summary of the quality and relevance of the review. These are held on a fully searchable database that is freely accessible (www.crd.york.ac.uk).

Economic evidence

As noted earlier, decision makers increasingly seek information on clinical *and* cost-effectiveness, in order to make optimal decisions about the use of limited healthcare resources. In parallel with the basic tenets of evidence-based practice, a framework has emerged to help users judge the quality and applicability of the results of economic studies that combine the clinical effectiveness of an interven-tion and the costs associated with its use.[50] The study designs that are used in eco-nomic evaluations are outlined in Box 3.2.

A ready source of economic evaluations that have been through a quality appraisal process is the National Health Service Economic Evaluations Database (NHS EED) – also produced by the Centre for Reviews and Dissemination at the University of York. Again, the research staff at this centre search for all economic evaluations related to healthcare and present them alongside a critical review judg-ing methodological rigour and relevance.[51]

Just as systematic reviews of randomized controlled trials are considered the highest-quality source of research evidence on the effectiveness of treatments, this method of data synthesis can also be applied to economic data. Reviews of economic data harness the same methods (PICO questions, comprehensive search strategies and quality appraisal), but use methods such as meta-analysis less often, since economic data do not readily lend themselves to this form of syn-thesis. Instead, data from a range of economic studies can be summarized visu-ally, using a permutation plot.[56,57,58] Briefly, the permutation plot presents nine

Box 3.2 Types of economic evaluations[51]

Full economic evaluations are studies in which a comparison of two or more interventions is undertaken and in which both the costs and outcomes of the alternatives are examined.

Cost–benefit analysis: Cost and outcomes are measured in monetary terms and the study calculates net monetary gains or losses (presented as a cost–benefit ratio). Increasingly used in calculating cost–benefit using the net benefit approach (see McCrone *et al.*[52] for an example).

Cost–effectiveness analysis: Compares interventions with a common or natural outcome (such as depression severity or depression-free days) to discover which produces the maximum outcome for the same input of resources in a given population (see Simon *et al.*[53] for an example).

Cost–utility analysis: Compares the benefits of alternative treatments by using utility measures such as quality-adjusted life years (QALYs) and may present relative costs per QALYs (see Pyne *et al.*[54] for an example).

Cost–minimization analysis: Assumes equal outcome for alternative treatments and describes which is associated with the lowest cost. Cost effectiveness analyses based on trials that demonstrate equivalent clinical outcomes are de facto cost minimization analyses (see Gask *et al.*[55] for an example).

possible outcomes, based on incremental effectiveness and costs (Figure 3.4). From an economic perspective, where the intervention increases clinical effectiveness at reduced cost, or increases cost with reduced clinical effectiveness, the decision to adopt or reject the intervention is simple. Unfortunately, such cases are rare. Much more prevalent are those where increased effectiveness is obtained at increased cost. Such studies raise difficult questions and require tough decisions about allocation of resources, because from an economic perspective the increased effectiveness comes at a cost, and paying that cost means that other services may not be funded (a so-called 'opportunity cost'). The permutation plot allows identification of the different combinations of effectiveness and cost, although it should be noted that it is a simplification of the complexities around the interpretation of cost data, and more sophisticated models are increasingly used.[59,60,61]

Methods used in the reviews

Search strategies

Systematic reviews often involve significant research funding and use a large group of researchers. Much of the resource is often used in developing a very comprehensive search strategy and checking thousands of studies and abstracts to identify papers. Such searches are beyond the scope of this book. To identify studies for the present reviews, published systematic reviews by the authors or others were taken

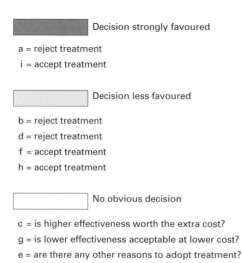

Effectiveness

Costs		Lower	Equal	Higher
	Higher	a	b	c
	Equal	d	e	f
	Lower	g	h	i

Decision strongly favoured

a = reject treatment
i = accept treatment

Decision less favoured

b = reject treatment
d = reject treatment
f = accept treatment
h = accept treatment

No obvious decision

c = is higher effectiveness worth the extra cost?
g = is lower effectiveness acceptable at lower cost?
e = are there any other reasons to adopt treatment?

Figure 3.4 Permutation matrix for possible outcomes of economic evaluations for study of intervention versus comparison.[42]

as the primary source of studies.[62–68] The relevant diagrams indicating the searches can be found in those publications. These initial lists of studies were then updated where necessary.

Data extraction and quality assessment

For the meta-analysis, a rating of overall methodological quality of randomized trials was based on two procedures designed to preserve group comparability: concealment of allocation and attrition.[9,69] Study quality was rated 'high' if allocation was adequately concealed (by central randomization or techniques such as the use of sealed, opaque envelopes),[49] and at least 80% of the randomized patients were followed up. Study quality was rated as 'medium' if one of these criteria was met, and 'low' if neither was met.

Analysis

Where possible, analyses of the effect of the different models on depression were divided into short-term outcomes (less than 12 months post-randomization) and long-term outcomes (12 months or more). The outcome measures in the studies included a mix of dichotomous (i.e. 'recovered' and 'not recovered') and continuous (i.e. number of depressive symptoms) measures. Continuous measures were used to compute an effect size (as described earlier in Box 3.1). Outcomes reported as dichotomous variables were translated to comparable effect sizes using the logit transformation.[44] Heterogeneity was measured using the I^2 statistic, and the pooling of studies used random-effects models. Economic analyses were synthesized using the 'permutation plot'.

Scope of the included studies

Many guidelines include evidence on the effectiveness of treatments tested in contexts very different from those in which the treatments are to be used. Often this is done for very good reasons, such as a desire to maximize use of the available evidence. It also may reflect a belief that certain disorders (such as depression) and psychological processes (such as those underlying psychological therapy) endure across different contexts.

A number of recent studies have explored the degree to which these contextual issues impact on the effectiveness of treatments. Raine and colleagues found that treatments for common somatic symptoms conducted in primary care generally reported smaller effects than those conducted in specialist care,[70] a result replicated in another review of psychological therapies for depression.[65] Churchill and colleagues found that psychological treatment for depression conducted on populations recruited outside clinical settings (such as volunteer populations) was also associated with higher effects.[71]

It is not known why effects may be smaller in primary care. It may reflect the lower severity of patients in this setting (such that patients in the control group tend to show high levels of spontaneous improvement), different types of problems or patients with different attitudes to treatment. It may reflect less specialized practitioners or shorter treatments. It may also reflect differences in study design (for example, the increased use of 'pragmatic' designs in the primary care setting).

Whatever the reason, the data suggest that considerable caution needs to be exercised when generalizing the results of data outside primary care. For this reason, the current analyses are restricted to patients recruited in primary care.

Access, equity and patient-centredness

In Chapter 1, we presented a framework for exploring the policy goals of different models. Issues of effectiveness and efficiency have been dealt with in the preceding chapter through analyses of clinical and cost effectiveness in trials and reviews. Randomized trials are often not effective vehicles for looking at these other policy goals. Trials can be conducted to look at access and equity issues. This involves defining a population of interest, and exploring the effects of an intervention on the proportion of patients who receive effective treatment, and the characteristics of those patients receiving care. For example, using an education and training model might mean that more patients in the population receive care, and that underserved groups (for example, ethnic minorities or those living in deprived circumstances) might be more likely to receive care than is usually the case. However, this design is rarely used, and most analyses of access and equity are indirect, describing the types of patient included in trials and the potential improvement in access associated with more efficient treatments, without providing a rigorous test of these benefits.

Issues of patient-centredness can be more easily explored either through outcome measures that take account of satisfaction and patient experience or by including measures of the 'worth' of the process of care in an economic analysis.[72] However, the technology for standardizing such assessments so that they can be compared across different interventions is at a rudimentary stage, and currently measures of patient experience are not generally given the same weight as issues of clinical and cost effectiveness in decision making.

Concluding comments

The framework of evidence-based practice serves as a framework for the rest of this book, and we will judge the effectiveness and cost effectiveness of each of the models of depression care in subsequent chapters using this framework.

REFERENCES

1 Sackett D, Rosenberg W, Gray J, Haynes B, Richardson W. Evidence-based medicine: what it is and what it is not. *British Medical Journal* 1996;312:71–2.
2 Sackett D, Wennberg J. Choosing the best research design for each question: it's time to stop squabbling over the 'best' methods. *British Medical Journal* 1997;315:1–2.
3 Maynard A. Evidence-based medicine: an incomplete method for informing treatment choices. *Lancet* 1997;349:126–8.
4 Drummond M, Stoddart G, Torrance G. *Methods for the Economic Evaluation of Health Care Programmes.* Oxford: Oxford Medical Publications, 1997.
5 Bower P, King M. Randomised controlled trials and the evaluation of psychological therapy. In: N Rowland, S Goss, editors. *Evidence-Based Counselling and Psychological Therapies.* London: Routledge, 2000;79–110.
6 Bower P. Efficacy in evidence-based practice. *Clinical Psychology and Psychotherapy* 2003;10:328–36.
7 Cook T, Campbell D. *Quasi-experimentation – Design and Analysis Issues for Field Settings.* Chicago: Rand McNally, 1979.
8 Kleijnen J, Gotzsche P, Kunz R, Oxman A, Chalmers I. So what's so special about randomisation? In: A Maynard, I Chalmers, editors. *Non-random Reflections on Health Services Research.* London: BMJ Publishing Group, 1997;93–106.

9 Schulz K, Chalmers I, Hayes R, Altman D. Empirical evidence of bias: dimensions of methodological quality associated with estimates of treatment effects in controlled trials. *Journal of the American Medical Association* 1995;273:408–12.

10 Altman D, Schulz K. Concealing treatment allocation in randomised trials. *British Medical Journal* 2001;323:446–7.

11 Schulz K, Grimes D. Allocation concealment in randomised trials: defending against deciphering. *Lancet* 2002;359:614–18.

12 Lipsey M. *Design Sensitivity: Statistical Power for Experimental Research*. Newbury Park, CA: Sage, 1990.

13 Hansen N, Lambert M. Clinical significance: an overview of methods. *Journal of Mental Health* 1996;5:17–24.

14 Ogles B, Lunnen K, Bonesteel K. Clinical significance: history, application and current practice. *Clinical Psychology Review* 2001;21:421–46.

15 Bower P, Wilson S, Mathers N. How often do UK primary care trials face recruitment delays? *Family Practice* 2007;24:601–3.

16 McDonald A, Knight R, Campbell M *et al*. What influences recruitment to randomised controlled trials? A review of trials funded by two UK funding agencies. *Trials* 2006;7:9

17 Torgerson D. Contamination in trials: is cluster randomisation the answer? *British Medical Journal* 2001;322:355–7.

18 Campbell M, Grimshaw J. Cluster randomised trials: time for improvement. *British Medical Journal* 1998;317:1171

19 Kerry S, Bland M. Trials which randomise practices I: how should they be analysed? *Family Practice* 1998;15:80–3.

20 Kerry S, Bland M. Trials which randomise practices II: sample size. *Family Practice* 1998;15:84–7.

21 Eldridge S, Ashby D, Feder G. Informed patient consent to participation in cluster randomized controlled trials: an empirical exploration of trials in primary care. *Clinical Trials* 2005;2:91–8.

22 Edwards S, Braunholtz D, Lilford R, Stevens A. Ethical issues in the design and conduct of cluster randomised controlled trials. *British Medical Journal* 1999;318:1407–9.

23 Hollis S, Campbell F. What is meant by intention to treat analysis? Survey of published randomised controlled trials. *British Medical Journal* 1999;319:670–4.

24 Schulz K, Grimes D. Sample size slippages in randomised trials: exclusions and the lost and wayward. *Lancet* 2002;359:781–5.

25 Crow R, Gage H, Hampson S, Hart J, Kimber A, Thomas H. The role of expectancies in the placebo effect and their use in the delivery of health care: a systematic review. *Health Technology Assessment* 1999;3:1–96.

26 Schulz K, Grimes D. Blinding in randomised trials: hiding who got what. *Lancet* 2002;359:696–700.

27 Campbell D. Relabeling internal and external validity for applied social scientists. In: W Trochim, editor. *Advances in Quasi-Experimental Design and Analysis*. San Francisco, CA: Jossey-Bass, 1986;67–77.

28 Shadish W, Matt G, Navarro A, Philips G. The effects of psychological therapies under clinically representative conditions: a meta-analysis. *Psychological Bulletin* 2000;126:512–19.

29 Weisz J, Weiss B, Donneberg G. The lab versus the clinic: effects of child and adolescent psychotherapy. *American Psychologist* 1992;47:1578–85.

30 Clarke G. Improving the transition from basic efficacy research to effectiveness studies: methodological issues and procedures. *Journal of Consulting and Clinical Psychology* 1995;63:718–25.

31 Schwartz D, Lellouch J. Explanatory and pragmatic attitudes in therapeutic trials. *Journal of Chronic Diseases* 1967;20:637–48.

32 Roland M, Torgerson D. What are pragmatic trials? *British Medical Journal* 1998;316:285.

33 Roberts C, Torgerson D. Baseline imbalance in randomised controlled trials. *British Medical Journal* 1999;319:185.

34 Mulrow C. Rationale for systematic reviews. *British Medical Journal* 1994;309:597–9.

35 Mulrow C. The medical review article: state of the science. *Annals of Internal Medicine* 1987;106:485–8.

36 Haynes B, McKibbon K, Wilczynski N, Walter S, Werre S, HEDGES team. Optimal search strategies for retrieving scientifically strong studies of treatment from Medline: analytical survey. *British Medical Journal* 2005;330:68–73.

37 Song F, Eastwood A, Gilbody S, Duley L, Sutton A. Publication and related biases. *Health Technology Assessment* 2000;4:1–115.

38 Juni P, Altman D, Egger M. Assessing the quality of controlled clinical trials. *British Medical Journal* 2001;323:42–6.

39 Sutton A, Abrams K, Jones D, Sheldon T, Song F. Systematic reviews of trials and other studies. *Health Technology Assessment* 1998;2:1–272.

40 Smith M, Glass G, Miller T. *The Benefits of Psychotherapy*. Baltimore, MD: Johns Hopkins University Press, 1980.

41 Beck A, Steer R, Brown G. *Manual for Beck Depression Inventory-II (BDI-II)*. San Antonia, TX: Psychological Corporation, 1996.

42 Cohen J. *Statistical Power Analysis for the Behavioural Sciences (2nd edition)*. New Jersey: Lawrence Erlbaum, 1988.

43 Lipsey M, Wilson D. The efficacy of psychological, educational and behavioural treatment. *American Psychologist* 1993;48:1181–209.

44 Lipsey M, Wilson D. *Practical Meta-Analysis*. Newbury Park, CA: Sage, 2001.

45 Hedges L, Olkin I. *Statistical Methods for Meta-Analysis*. London: Academic Press, 1985.

46 Ekers D, Richards D, Gilbody S. A meta-analysis of randomized trials of behavioural treatment of depression. *Psychological Medicine* 2008;38:611–23.

47 Higgins J, Thompson S, Deeks J, Altman D. Statistical heterogeneity in systematic reviews of clinical trials: a critical appraisal of guidelines and practice. *Journal of Health Services Research and Policy* 2002;7:51–61.

48 Higgins J, Thompson S, Deeks J, Altman D. Measuring inconsistency in meta-analyses. *British Medical Journal* 2003;327:557–60.

49 Higgins J, Green S. *Cochrane Handbook for Systematic Reviews of Interventions Version 5.0.1*. Cochrane Collaboration, 2009. Available at: www.cochrane-handbook.org.

50 Drummond M, Jefferson T. Guidelines for authors and peer reviewers of economic submissions to the BMJ. *British Medical Journal* 1996;313:275–83.

51 NHS Centre for Reviews and Dissemination. *Making Cost Effectiveness Information Available: the NHS Economic Evaluation Database project (CRD report 6)*. York, UK: University of York, 2001.

52 McCrone P, Knapp M, Proudfoot J *et al*. Cost effectiveness of computerised cognitive-behavioural therapy for anxiety and depression in primary care: randomised controlled trial. *British Journal of Psychiatry* 2004;185:55–62.

53 Simon G, Katon W, Von Korff M *et al.* Cost-effectiveness of a collaborative care program for primary care patients with persistent depression. *American Journal of Psychiatry* 2001;158:1638–44.

54 Pyne J, Rost K, Zhang M, Williams K, Smith J, Fortney J. Cost-effectiveness of a primary care depression intervention. *Journal of General Internal Medicine* 2003;18:432–41.

55 Gask L, Dowrick C, Dixon C *et al.* A pragmatic cluster randomized controlled trial of an educational intervention for GPs in the assessment and management of depression. *Psychological Medicine* 2004;34:63–72.

56 Birch S, Gaffni A. Cost effectiveness and cost utility analyses: methods for the non economic evaluation of healthcare programs and how we can do better. In: E Geisler, O Heller, editors. *Managing Technology in Healthcare*. Norwell, MA: Kluwer Academic, 1996.

57 Black W. The CE plane: a graphic representation of cost effectiveness. *Medical Decision Making* 1990;10:21–4.

58 Nixon J, Khan K, Kleijnen J. Summarising economic evaluations in systematic reviews: a new approach. *British Medical Journal* 2001;322:1596–8.

59 Fenwick E, Claxton K, Sculpher M. Representing uncertainty: the role of cost-effectiveness acceptability curves. *Health Economics* 2002;10:779–87.

60 Fenwick E, O'Brien B, Briggs A. Cost-effectiveness acceptability curves – facts, fallacies and frequenctly asked questions. *Health Economics* 2004;13:405–15.

61 Fenwick E, Byford S. A guide to cost-effectiveness acceptability curves. *The British Journal of Psychiatry* 2005;187:106–8.

62 Gilbody S, Bower P, Fletcher J, Richards D, Sutton A. Collaborative care for depression: a systematic review and cumulative meta-analysis. *Archives of Internal Medicine* 2006;166:2314–21.

63 Gilbody S, Whitty P, Grimshaw J, Thomas R. Educational and organisational interventions to improve the management of depression in primary care: a systematic review. *Journal of the American Medical Association* 2003;289:3145–51.

64 Harkness E, Bower P. On-site mental health workers delivering psychological therapy and psychosocial interventions to patients in primary care: effects on the professional practice of primary care providers. *Cochrane Database of Systematic Reviews* 2009;Issue 1:CD000532. DOI: 10.1002/14651858.CD000532.pub2.

65 Cuijpers P, Van Straten A, van Schaik A, Andersson G. Psychological treatment of depression in primary care: a meta-analysis. *British Journal of General Practice* 2009;59:51–60.

66 National Institute for Health and Clinical Excellence. *Depression: the Treatment and Management of Depression in Adults (update)*. London: National Institute for Health and Clinical Excellence, 2009. Available at: www.nice.org.uk/nicemedia/pdf/Depression_Update_FULL_GUIDELINE.pdf

67 Bower P, Rowland N. Effectiveness and cost effectiveness of counselling in primary care. *Cochrane Database of Systematic Reviews* 2006;Issue 3:CD001025. DOI: 10.1002/14651858.CD001025.pub2.

68 Cape J, Whittington C, Buszewicz M, Wallace P, Underwood L. Effectiveness of brief psychological therapies for anxiety and depression in primary care: meta-analysis and meta-regression. *BMC Health Services Research* 2010;8:39.

69 Dumville J, Torgerson D, Hewitt C. Reporting attrition in randomised controlled trials. *British Medical Journal* 2006;332:969–71.

70 Raine R, Haines A, Sensky T, Hutchings A, Larkin K, Black N. Systematic review of mental health interventions for patients with common somatic symptoms: can research

evidence from secondary care be extrapolated to primary care? *British Medical Journal* 2002;325:1082

71 Churchill R, Hunot V, Corney R *et al.* A systematic review of controlled trials of the effectiveness and cost-effectiveness of brief psychological treatments for depression. *Health Technology Assessment* 2001;5:1–173.

72 Donaldson C, Shackley P. Does 'process utility' exist? a case study of willingness to pay for laparoscopic cholecystectomy. *Social Science and Medicine* 1997;44:699–707.

4

Anatomy of a review

Peter Bower and Simon Gilbody

Although the principles of systematic reviews are fundamentally quite simple, the application of these principles is often difficult. In this chapter we seek to provide practical examples of many of the core review processes outlined in Chapter 3, to help the reader appreciate the challenges of applying these techniques in practice.

We will start with the process of developing a systematic review question and appropriate inclusion and exclusion criteria, outline the strategies used in developing a search, and then focus down on the detailed data extraction from an exemplar randomized controlled trial for quality appraisal and meta-analysis.

Developing the research question

As noted in Chapter 3, research questions underlying systematic reviews are often based on the PICO formula: Population, Intervention, Comparison, Outcome. For the purposes of the book, our core question is 'What is the best model for the delivery of care for depression?'. This question lacks specificity, so we will need to use the PICO formula to provide a more precise version. We have outlined our four models previously, so we now have four PICO questions, which have the same structure:

In patients with depression [Population], is education and training [Intervention] more effective than usual care [Comparison] in reducing depression [Outcome]?

The other three questions are the same, but with the Intervention modified to read 'consultation-liaison', 'collaborative care' and 'referral'. These are our primary questions, although an additional issue clearly relates to the relative effectiveness of the different models.

Although those questions provide a better basis for our review, there are still major ambiguities that we would need to clarify, by developing more specific inclusion and exclusion criteria to go with the PICO. For example, 'in patients with

Depression in Primary Care: Evidence and Practice, ed. Simon Gilbody and Peter Bower. Published by Cambridge University Press. © Cambridge University Press 2011.

depression' has a number of possible interpretations. It might be restricted to those formally diagnosed with depression by a research psychiatrist within the trial. This has the advantage of ensuring that all patients entering the trial have the same core diagnosis. However, a trial might include patients who receive a 'clinical' diagnosis from their usual health professional. Such diagnoses are less standardized and more likely to include misdiagnoses (which might threaten internal validity) but better represent the reality of depression treatment in the community (increasing external validity). Equally, patients who have symptoms of depression but who have not received a diagnosis (so-called subthreshold disorders – see Chapter 1) might also be included.

Each of these approaches is legitimate, because there is still no consensus about the best way to understand depression,[1,2,3] and different decision makers may have different views on this issue and different needs. Reviews that use different criteria at this stage will potentially include different studies and come up with very different results, despite all ostensibly assessing 'depression'. In one sense it is less important to determine which approach is right or wrong and more important to identify the impact of the different decisions on the content and the results of the review.

Similar issues are raised in relation to 'Intervention'. Although we propose that the four models discussed in Chapter 2 are qualitatively different, there are significant 'grey' areas, and even if there is agreement about the models, the precise definition of each is complex. For example, there are major controversies over the definition and labelling of different psychological therapies, and there may be debates over the training and background needed to meet that definition.[4] For example, if a general practitioner (GP) in the context of a trial receives a short training course over two days in counselling skills, is that enough for the study to be considered a study of 'psychological therapy'? Possibly not, but if that course was over two years, would the study then be included or excluded?

The issues are magnified in the context of something like 'collaborative care'.[5] This is by definition a 'complex intervention' (see Chapter 2) where the exact ingredients are difficult to specify.[6] Published reviews differ markedly in the studies that are included and excluded.[7,8,9] Again, this is all part of legitimate difference of scientific opinion.

Systematic reviews are designed to be as clear and explicit as possible, but it is unlikely that this will remove ambiguity and disagreement entirely. One way of making the cause of disagreements clear is to have a 'table of excluded studies', which details studies that appear eligible but have been excluded on the basis of certain criteria. Such tables can take up a lot of space, which is why they are often found in online publications such as Cochrane reviews rather than paper journals.

The criteria for 'Comparators' and 'Outcomes' also need to be specified, but these are often less tightly defined. There is no reason why a review cannot included a range of comparators: for example, a review of psychological therapy could compare that treatment with no treatment, usual care arms, other psychological therapies and other treatments (such as medication). All could reasonably be included in a review, although it is good to (a) specify a list of comparators in advance and (b) specify how they will be combined or distinguished. For example, a review might compare psychological therapy against a range of 'no treatment' comparators, such as no treatment, usual care and waiting lists. These are not identical, and it is possible that each control group has a different effect on patient outcomes, but it would reasonable to combine them in the same analysis, and many reviews take that approach. It would be more contentious to combine studies that used usual care and 'active treatment' comparators such as medication (see Chapter 3).

Similarly, a review can include a wide range of outcomes.[4,10–13] For the purposes of the analyses presented in this book, we have focused on depression and costs, as these are often of greatest interest to decision makers. However, there are a range of other outcomes which could be included, such as patient satisfaction and other measures of patient-centredness, equity and access measures, and other types of outcomes such as social function, disability and quality of life. Generally these will be analysed separately (indeed, different measures of outcome from the same study cannot be combined in the same meta-analysis), but the review will be more comprehensive if all are included in separate analyses within the same review. However, some reviews identify a 'primary' outcome, which is the one that will receive most attention in reporting and the one on which the treatment is meant to be judged. The list of other outcomes would then be considered 'secondary', providing additional supporting evidence about the effectiveness of the treatment.

Developing a comprehensive search

A comprehensive search is the hallmark of a systematic review. There are many ways of searching for studies, including checking previous published reviews, contacting subject experts and hand searching, which involves 'a manual page-by-page examination of the entire contents of a journal issue to identify all eligible reports of trials'.[14] However, the main focus of a systematic review is usually on the electronic database search, and that is what we will concentrate on here.

The basis of the search is the PICO formula, as that provides details of the core criteria of studies that the search will try to identify. The next step is to translate some or all of the PICO into specific search terms. There are two broad types of search term. Standardized *subject headings* (called MeSH terms in MEDLINE) are the result of an indexing process by the publishers, where labels are attached to papers as they are entered on the database. *Text terms* are the words and phrases that are part of the actual text of the paper (where the text may be restricted to the title and the abstract, or may include the full text). Although there can be a lot of overlap between these search terms in the papers that they identify, they are not identical. Subject headings tend to be more precise, and have the advantage that they are standardized, so that a subject heading may be added by the indexers to two papers even if the authors of the individual papers have not used the same terms in their paper. However, a good search will use both approaches. Each search has to be customized for the various databases that are available to the review team.

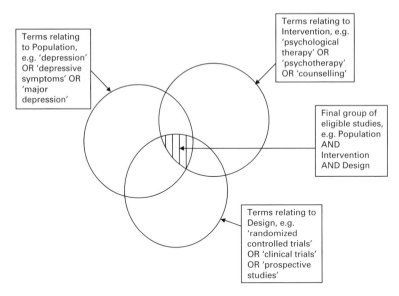

Figure 4.1 **Structure of a search using the PICO formula.**

The idea behind a search is to find the right trade-off between *sensitivity* and *specificity*. Sensitivity refers to the ability of the search to identify all relevant studies. Adding search terms and using very broad terms increases sensitivity. But the downside is that this reduces specificity, which is the ability of the search to screen out irrelevant studies. Different searches will make different trade-offs, and this often relates to the resources available.

Not all elements of the PICO have to be entered in the search. Terms for Population and Intervention are almost always included (Figure 4.1), and are often combined with a range of terms for the study designs to be included in the review (for example, if the review is to be restricted to randomized controlled trials). If a review included a range of comparators and a range of outcomes (see above), it is not always necessary to include them in a search. For example, if a reviewer wants to find all the collaborative care studies in depressed patients, but is interested in all outcomes of such studies, it is easier to design a search that identifies all studies of collaborative care studies in depression, and then identify the various outcomes by reading the papers after the database search has been completed.

Each database has a particular vocabulary and structure for the search, but some terms are common, for example those used to combine searches. Terms within one aspect of the PICO (for example, all the terms relating to Population) are combined using the OR term, which adds the results of individual searches together, bringing together papers that meet *any* of the search criteria. Finally, terms relating to different aspects of the PICO (such as Population and Intervention) are then combined using the AND term, which identifies only those papers that meet *all* criteria (i.e. include terms relating to Population *and* Intervention).

Figure 4.2 shows aspects of a complex search used to identify trials of education and training for depression, from a published review,[15] and highlights the

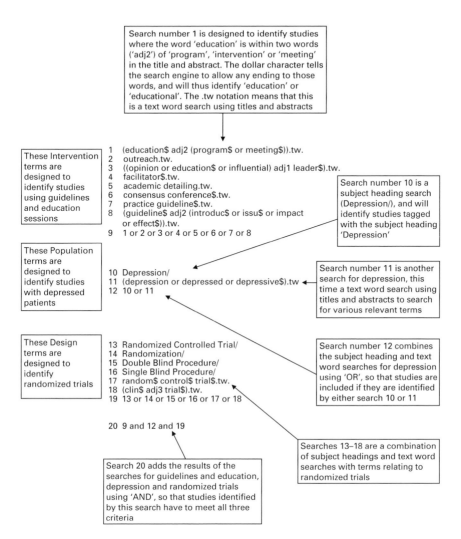

Search number 1 is designed to identify studies where the word 'education' is within two words ('adj2') of 'program', 'intervention' or 'meeting' in the title and abstract. The dollar character tells the search engine to allow any ending to those words, and will thus identify 'education' or 'educational'. The .tw notation means that this is a text word search using titles and abstracts

These Intervention terms are designed to identify studies using guidelines and education sessions

1   (education$ adj2 (program$ or meeting$)).tw.
2   outreach.tw.
3   ((opinion or education$ or influential) adj1 leader$).tw.
4   facilitator$.tw.
5   academic detailing.tw.
6   consensus conference$.tw.
7   practice guideline$.tw.
8   (guideline$ adj2 (introduc$ or issu$ or impact or effect$)).tw.
9   1 or 2 or 3 or 4 or 5 or 6 or 7 or 8

Search number 10 is a subject heading search (Depression/), and will identify studies tagged with the subject heading 'Depression'

These Population terms are designed to identify studies with depressed patients

10 Depression/
11 (depression or depressed or depressive$).tw
12 10 or 11

Search number 11 is another search for depression, this time a text word search using titles and abstracts to search for various relevant terms

These Design terms are designed to identify randomized trials

13 Randomized Controlled Trial/
14 Randomization/
15 Double Blind Procedure/
16 Single Blind Procedure/
17 random$ control$ trial$.tw.
18 (clin$ adj3 trial$).tw.
19 13 or 14 or 15 or 16 or 17 or 18

Search number 12 combines the subject heading and text word searches for depression using 'OR', so that studies are included if they are identified by either search 10 or 11

20 9 and 12 and 19

Searches 13–18 are a combination of subject headings and text word searches with terms relating to randomized trials

Search 20 adds the results of the searches for guidelines and education, depression and randomized trials using 'AND', so that studies identified by this search have to meet all three criteria

Figure 4.2 Extracts from a search for education and training studies.[4]

combinations of PICO criteria, text terms and subject headings, and their combinations through AND/OR terms.

Generating a good search strategy takes time and experimentation, and each will require modification to work on each specific database. Often searches will pick up too many 'hits' (i.e. identify too many studies), which cannot possibly be checked within the resources available to the research team. Decisions then have to be made on ways to cut down the search. This may involve removing terms, or placing other limits on the search, i.e. only searching for studies after a certain date, or excluding studies in languages other than English. The potential for bias in such decisions is clear, and would need to be considered in the discussion of any review, although little is known about the trade-offs.[16] To develop searches, it is best to enlist the help of a specialist librarian, but it is also useful to access publicly available reviews (such as those on the *Cochrane Library*) as these provide their full search strategies, which can be used as the basis for new searches.

Once the list of studies has been identified from the searches, these must be checked for eligibility, optimally by two researchers working independently. The first stage involves checking the title and abstracts. No matter how good the search, the bulk of studies identified will not be relevant for various reasons. Many can be rejected on the basis of the title alone, whereas others will be rejected on the basis of the detail provided in the abstract. Finally, some papers will have to be read in their entirety to make a decision about their inclusion. There are likely to be disagreements among the researchers about the inclusion and exclusion of papers. These are best resolved through discussion with a wider team or independent third party. The search process should be fully documented using the PRISMA standard (see Chapter 3).[17]

As noted above, studies that fail to meet the criteria should be documented in an 'excluded studies table'. There is no agreed rule about the studies that should be included in this table, although clearly this does not relate to the many thousands that are rejected at the early stages of the search when titles and abstracts are examined. A good rule of thumb is that the excluded studies table should include those studies that meet some but not all of the criteria, and which experts in the area might have expected to see in the review.[14] By listing them in the excluded studies table and providing a reason for their exclusion, the reviewers can reassure the reader that they have not missed those studies, and that they have been excluded on the basis of explicit, predefined criteria, and not because their results somehow do not fit the researchers' preconceptions.

Extracting data and appraising the quality of study design

For the purposes of example, we will use a study published by the UK Health Technology Assessment Programme, conducted by Simpson and colleagues, entitled 'A randomised controlled trial to evaluate the effectiveness and cost-effectiveness of counselling patients with chronic depression'.[18] This trial is clearly relevant to the questions posed in this book about the effectiveness of different models, as the counselling intervention is an example of the 'referral' model, and the trial takes place in the primary care setting and involves patients with depression. The Health Technology Assessment Programme also publishes freely available reports on its trials, which can be downloaded from its website (www.hta.ac.uk).

The process of *data extraction* involves recording data from published reports of trials, in a form that is accurate, accessible and useful to readers. Accuracy is ensured by using multiple independent researchers to conduct extraction where possible. Accessibility and utility requires extracting data from the report, summarizing and presenting it in a form that does not simply repeat the data already presented, but seeks to present it in a way that allows the reader to rapidly understand the nature of the trial and, more importantly, to compare the different trials in a review on core characteristics.

Data extraction usually involves development of a form with headings that relate to key aspects of the trial. Headings will generally be grouped according to the PICO, but with more detail relating to the precise nature of the individual trial. For example, details of the Population part of the PICO will have data on the type of depression in the patient population, together with data on patient characteristics (e.g. age, sex and ethnicity) and key inclusion and exclusion criteria used in the trial.

The purpose of data extraction is to produce a useful and succinct overview of studies in a way that conveys important detail without reproducing the whole of a paper in a different format. The actual level of detail involved in data extraction varies widely. In the examples provided in this book, we have taken a limited approach because of the space issues. Online publications such as the *Cochrane Library* and journal e-supplements allow a far greater level of detail.

Data from individual studies are generally extracted into a series of tables. Again, the number of tables will depend on the nature of the review, but it is common to provide a table detailing characteristics of the Population, one on the Intervention (often combined with data on the Comparison), one on Design and quality criteria, and possibly one detailing the outcome measures and a narrative description of the results (depending in part on whether a meta-analysis is planned).

The process of data extraction is often an iterative one. Initially, the data extracted may be recorded directly from the text of the paper. However, because of the variability in how that information is presented, modifications will be required as additional studies are added, to ensure that the reader can quickly and efficiently make comparisons *between* studies. This will sometimes require recalculation of data, to ensure it is presented in the same way. For example, some studies will provide data on the percentage of females in the trial, while others will provide data on the percentage of males. It is helpful if the data are presented in the same form to ensure that rapid comparisons can be made easily and accurately. Some of the data extracted will relate to planned aspects of the study (e.g. inclusion criteria will relate to the types of patient that the study wished to recruit, or the length of treatment that was planned to be provided), whereas other data will relate to what actually happened (e.g. the actual severity of depression in the patients recruited, and the actual length of treatments that were received).

Reviewers will often add columns to the data extraction table with codes that they might find useful in the review. For example, one column might have details of how depression was defined in the particular study, while the next column might then apply a code to identify the methods used in terms of a small number of core categories. For example, the specific detail might state 'Patients with significant depression symptoms identified on the basis of screening in the waiting room using a self-report depression screening questionnaire (the Patient Health Questionnaire 9)'. The reviewer might then add one or more codes to identify the methods used for recruitment in this study (i.e. 'screening', compared with 'recruitment by a clinician') and the method of definition of depression (i.e. 'depressive symptoms', compared with a 'research diagnosis'). When it comes to ratings of the quality of the study, reviewers often add a simple code to indicate whether a quality criterion was met (e.g. 'Done' or 'Not done' for allocation concealment). The exact codes used will depend on the particular interests of the reviewer and the sorts of issues that they think are important.

The following pages show exemplar data extraction tables for the Simpson trial. Core data has been extracted, but decisions have to be made about what to extract, as the report is very detailed. The key issue is that the data extraction process is meant to help the reader make comparisons between studies in terms of key characteristics. There is little point in slavishly extracting every bit of detail, because the tables will be unwieldy and will overwhelm the reader. It makes more sense to extract data that are highly pertinent to the particular questions that the review is designed to answer, and then highlight those characteristics where most studies report data (so that comparisons can be made). As we intend to explore data through meta-analysis, no table has been created for the results.

The report of the Simpson trial provides a lot of detail about the patients in the study, some of which has been extracted into the tables (see Table 4.1). Most depression trials in the UK do not recruit significant numbers of patients from ethnic minorities for various reasons, but no data were presented on this issue. However, the rest of the report has highly detailed information on clinical and demographic characteristics of patients.

Similarly, the report also provides detailed information on aspects of the treatment (Table 4.2). Indeed, the level of detail concerning the background and experience of the therapists presented in the report is too much for a table of this kind, and needs careful summary.

Table 4.3 details information about study design and quality. As noted in Chapter 3, allocation concealment is a critical factor in trials, and in this study the procedure was done by an independent member of the health authority. This ensured allocation concealment (as the person who judged the patient's eligibility was separate from the randomization process).

The study used a sample size calculation to determine the number of patients needed. It is possible to interpret the power analysis in terms of the effect size calculations outlined in Chapter 3. The study was powered to detect a difference of 3.5 points on the Beck Depression Inventory, assuming a standard deviation of 8. In effect size terms, this is an effect of 0.44 (3.5 divided by 8), which is approximately a 'medium' effect. Therefore, the study had sufficient patients and power to detect a 'medium' effect of counselling on depressive symptoms, should one exist. If the actual effect of counselling was 'large', the study would also be adequately powered, but if the effect was 'small', the sample size would be too small to detect that reliably. By setting these parameters, the authors suggest that 'small' effects are not of interest to them.

The report provides data on baseline comparability, together with statistical tests of those differences. As noted in Chapter 3, such tests are not always appropriate, and whatever the results of the tests, it is worth checking the magnitude of any differences. As can be seen in the report, the proportion of married patients is very similar (63% in the intervention and 67% in the control), and the data also demonstrate good comparability on proportions with children, patients' housing

Table 4.1 Exemplar data extraction table for Population for Simpson trial[18]

Population	Recruitment method	Inclusion criteria	Exclusion criteria	Depression characteristics	Age and sex	Ethnicity	Other characteristics
Patients with depression or depression/anxiety as their main symptom for over 6 months	GP referral initially, then waiting room screening after recruitment difficulties	Aged 18–70 Mild to moderate symptoms of depression for 6+ months Depression or depression/ anxiety as main symptom Score of 14+ on Beck Depression Inventory	Severe depression or anxiety Symptoms of anxiety only History of substance abuse or psychosis History of suicide attempts Chronic depression (5+ years) Frequent attenders with unexplainable physical symptoms Receipt of counselling in last 6 months	Mean Beck Depression Inventory scores 21.5 (intervention), 19.8 (control) Proportion of patients with mild depression 30% (intervention) 44% (control) Moderate depression 34% (intervention) 29% (control) Severe depression 36% (intervention) 27% (control)	Mean age 42 (intervention) and 44 (control) 80% female	No data	Married (65%), separated or divorced (16%), single (11%), widowed (8%)

Table 4.2 Exemplar data extraction table for Intervention and Comparison for Simpson trial[18]

Intervention	Therapists	Treatment duration	Other interventions	Adherence	Comparator
Counselling 6 counsellors used a psychodynamic model and 2 a cognitive model No treatment manuals were used	8 counsellors (6 females and 2 males) All were accredited or eligible for accreditation from the key professional body All were trained and had experience of counselling in a general practice	6–12 sessions in line with local guidelines	Medical records indicated proportion of patients taking medication during trial: 43% (intervention) and 46% (control)	87% of those referred actually saw a counsellor at least once Mean number of sessions: 6 (range 1–16)	Usual care Only restriction placed was that they were not allowed to refer control patients to the counsellor

Table 4.3 Exemplar data extraction table for Design for Simpson trial[18]

Allocation concealment	Allocation concealment code	Sample size calculation	Comparability at baseline	Sample size and attrition	Attrition code	Outcome assessment
Details of patients who were appropriate and had agreed to take part were given by hand to the health authority that undertook the randomization, using random number tables	Done	Yes – to detect a difference in outcome between the groups of 3.5 (SD = 8) in Beck Depression Inventory score at 90% power and a 5% significance level, approximately 70–80 patients were required in each group	Differences in baseline Beck Depression Inventory scores approached statistical significance (mean intervention: 21.8; mean control: 19.8)	181 randomized 161 followed up at 6 months (89%) 143 followed up at 12 months (79%)	Done	Assessors potentially blind to allocation when conducting assessments

situation and employment. Patient ages were similar, but there were more men in the control group. Of greater concern is the fact that there was quite a large difference in baseline depression scores (a mean on the Beck Depression Inventory of 21.5 in the intervention group and 19.8 in the controls, a difference that was nearly statistically significant and equates to an 'effect size' of around 0.3, although that is a difference *prior to treatment*). Baseline measures of trial outcomes are almost always the best predictors of outcomes after treatment, so a difference here would be of concern. As noted in Chapter 3, baseline differences can emerge by chance alone (particularly in smaller trials) and this does not necessarily mean that randomization was in some way subverted. There are statistical methods of ameliorating this difference, and this sort of problem does not render a trial useless, but it should be noted as part of the quality assessment.

Data on the important issue of attrition are provided in a CONSORT diagram in the report, which indicates that 89% of patients were followed up at 6 months and 79% at 12 months. The CONSORT also breaks these data down by group, so that we can see that follow-up rates were 89% in both groups at 6 months, but were 82% in the intervention group and 76% in the control group at 12 months. Although there is some difference at 12 months between the groups in terms of the proportion of patients who remained in the study (i.e. *differential attrition*), the overall follow-up rate is high and the difference between groups relatively small.

The final issue concerns outcome assessments and blinding. Blinding patients to the intervention is not generally appropriate in a pragmatic trial and with an active intervention such as counselling. Due to the method of allocation concealment, the person doing the outcome assessment was not explicitly told which group the patient was in, and thus they were potentially blind to their allocation when the assessments were done. It is not clear how important this was though, as the outcome assessments were self-reported, and it is not clear whether patients broke that blinding by letting the assessor know whether they had received counselling or not.

Using the methods outlined at the end of Chapter 3, the trial would be given a 'high' rating for quality. This takes account of the allocation concealment and the follow-up rate of over 80%, but the quality rating system does ignore the issue identified earlier with baseline comparability. It should be noted that this would use the 6-month follow-up rate – at 12 months, the rate slips just below 80%. Attempting to simplify quality assessments through coding systems such as this necessarily requires arbitrary decisions.

The assessment of study quality within systematic reviews is subject to ongoing debate, and there are numerous approaches that can be used. In our approach in this book we have selected simple items of quality (randomization, concealment of allocation and attrition), since these have theoretical and empirical evidence to support their use.[19,20,21] Other approaches include more complex and lengthy lists of 'quality assessment items'. One frequently used approach is the Cochrane 'Assessment of Bias' tool, and interested readers are advised to consult the *Cochrane Handbook* for a further discussion of these issues.[14]

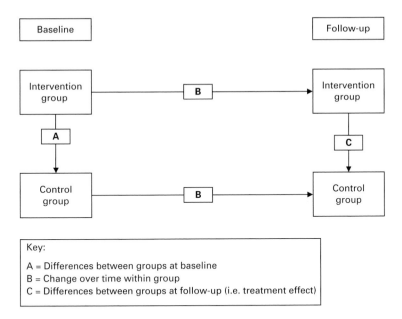

Figure 4.3 Analyses and comparisons in a trial.

Analysing outcome data

The abstract of the report indicates that:

There was an overall significant improvement in the actual scores over time but no difference between groups or between CBT [cognitive-behavioural therapy] and psychodynamic counselling approaches at either 6 or 12 months.

Trial results can be presented in various formats, which relate to different ways of looking at the data (Figure 4.3). When baseline and follow-up assessments are made, randomization is designed to ensure that the two groups are comparable at baseline assessment, and the core trial analysis looks at differences between mean scores at follow-up (*between groups*). The first line in the quote above also indicates that the changes over time in the groups were 'significant' (*within groups*). That is entirely legitimate, but this is an entirely different type of analysis that tells us nothing about the comparison. It is not legitimate to compare changes within groups (i.e. to compare the changes between baseline and follow-up of the intervention and the control group) and somehow make inferences about relative effectiveness of the interventions.

Narrative descriptions of results such as those reported above are common in reports of randomized trials, but are less useful for the systematic reviewer for several reasons. Firstly, the statement about 'statistical significance' is a categorical result (i.e. a treatment either does or does not demonstrate 'statistical significance'), but says nothing about the magnitude of the difference. Secondly, the results are not easily compared across studies, so that the reviewer cannot determine the

Table 4.4 Outcome data extraction table for the Simpson trial[18]

Outcome	Follow-up (months)	Intervention Mean, SD, n	Control Mean, SD, n	Mean difference	Pooled SD	Effect size	95% confidence interval
Beck Depression Inventory	6	16.0, 9.3, 82	16.0, 8.1, 79	0	8.7	0	−0.31 to 0.31
Beck Depression Inventory	12	15.0, 9.8, 75	15.3, 8.6, 68	−0.3	9.3	−0.03	−0.36 to 0.30
Brief Symptom Inventory	6	65.4, 9.7, 82	64.1, 9.3, 79	1.3	9.5	0.14	−0.17 to 0.45
Brief Symptom Inventory	12	64.1, 11.3, 75	64.0, 9.6, 68	0.1	10.5	0.01	−0.32 to 0.34
Inventory of Interpersonal Problems	6	41.3, 20.8, 82	37.8, 17.1, 79	3.5	19.1	0.18	−0.13 to 0.49
Inventory of Interpersonal Problems	12	40.2, 22.3, 75	38.2, 18.3, 68	2.0	20.5	0.10	−0.23 to 0.43
Social Adjustment Scale	6	2.4, 0.6, 82	2.4, 0.5, 79	0	0.6	0	−0.31 to 0.31
Social Adjustment Scale	12	2.3, 0.6, 75	2.4, 0.6, 68	−0.1	0.6	−0.17	−0.50 to 0.16

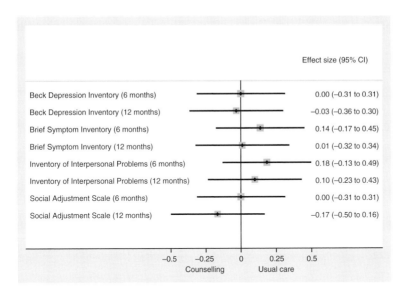

Figure 4.4 Effect size calculations for the Simpson study.

relative impact in this and other trials of the same treatment. To overcome these problems, we need to determine effect sizes (see Chapter 3).

The key to calculating an effect size is identifying the correct data. Many trials do not report any relevant data, and an effect size cannot be calculated. Other trials report some relevant data, and there are many different ways of determining an effect size from various presentations of data.[22] To calculate an effect size from continuous data, the reviewer is ideally looking for three pieces of data: the mean scores of the intervention and control group at follow-up, their respective standard deviations and group samples sizes.

The data from the Simpson study are presented in Table 4.4. Four outcome measures are available (the Beck Depression Inventory, Brief Symptom Inventory, Inventory of Interpersonal Problems and the Social Adjustment Scale). Each provides a different measure of dysfunction, although the primary outcome for this study was the Beck Depression Inventory. It is important to note that all these measures are scored such that a reduction in scores was an improvement. If scales are scored in the opposite direction, then the interpretation of their mean and the effect sizes must be appropriate.

Table 4.4 shows the raw data from the trial report, together with the mean difference (i.e. the intervention group mean minus the control group mean), the pooled standard deviation (a measure of the variability in outcomes, calculated over the two groups combined) and the effect size (the mean difference divided by the pooled standard deviation).

Note that the calculation of the effect size of the Beck Depression Inventory scores at 6 months is in some ways unnecessary: the mean difference is zero, so the effect size is also zero (although the calculation also provides a confidence interval, which gives us some idea of the precision of our estimate). It is important to note that this does not mean that patients do not get better, since both groups show reductions in scores from baseline. Instead, this means that those changes from baseline do not differ between groups, and that having counselling is not associated with bigger reductions than remaining in usual care (Figure 4.3).

The effect size of counselling on other measures and at other time points varies somewhat (Figure 4.4). The effect of counselling on the Brief Symptom Inventory and Inventory of Interpersonal Problems at 6 months approaches a 'small' effect size (although the data actually show a better impact on the control group, because the effect size is positive). The opposite is true on the Social Adjustment Scale at 12 months (where the benefit is associated with receiving counselling). However, none of the effects actually reach the 'small' effect size criteria, and thus our overall interpretation is that the trial shows no effect of counselling over usual care (at least in patients with chronic depression). Note also that the confidence intervals for the effect size estimates are very wide. For example, the confidence interval for the effect of counselling on the Social Adjustment Scale at 12 months includes both a 'medium' effect improvement associated with counselling (effect size –0.50) and a 'small' deterioration (effect size 0.16). This highlights that, although the trial was powered through a formal sample size calculation, the precision associated with the estimate of the trial is limited. One of the advantages of meta-analysis is overcoming this limitation.

What does effect size measurement add beyond the narrative of the results in the quote at the beginning of this section? In this case, the results agree, because a statistical test of 'no significant difference' is simply confirmed by the effect size data. However, the effect size data provide more detail about the magnitude and direction of the effects. It is also important to note that agreement between statistical significance and effect size estimates is not always the case. Where trials are very small, power can be limited (see Chapter 3), which means that a statistical test may report 'no significant difference' even when one exists, simply because the sample size is too small to detect an underlying difference. Alternatively, a trial with a much larger sample size may report a statistically significant difference that actually represents a very small effect size that is clinically trivial.

As shown in Table 4.4, if the right data are presented it is possible to calculate effect sizes for every outcome measure at every follow-up point. However, not all of these can be used in a meta-analysis, because each meta-analysis should include only one data point for each trial (although a review may include many separate meta-analyses). So in principle it would be acceptable to run separate meta-analyses of depression outcomes in the short term (6 months) and in the long term (12 months), and then run a separate meta-analysis for each of the other outcomes at each time point. However, the more data analyses are presented, the more confusing the results can be, which is why analysts often like to focus on one or two as 'primary' outcomes. For the purposes of the current book, we focus on depression outcomes alone.

There are additional complexities to take into account in effect size calculations. For example, modifications have to be made if a trial includes more than two arms, as well as taking account of cluster trials (see Chapter 3). These issues are beyond the scope of this book, and readers are encouraged to consult the *Cochrane Handbook* and other relevant texts.[14,22,23]

REFERENCES

1   Middleton H, Shaw I. Distinguishing mental illness in primary care. *British Medical Journal* 2000;320:1420–1.

2   Shorter E, Tyrer P. Separation of anxiety and depressive disorders: blind alley in psychopharmacology and classification of disease. *British Medical Journal* 2003;327:158–60.

3   Mirowsky J, Ross C. Psychiatric diagnosis as reified measurement. *Journal of Health and Social Behaviour* 1989;30:11–25.

4   Smith M, Glass G, Miller T. *The Benefits of Psychotherapy*. Baltimore, MD: Johns Hopkins University Press, 1980.

5   Bower P, Gilbody S, Richards D, Fletcher J, Sutton A. Collaborative care for depression in primary care. Making sense of a complex intervention: systematic review and meta regression. *British Journal of Psychiatry* 2006;189:484–93.

6   Campbell M, Fitzpatrick R, Haines A *et al*. Framework for design and evaluation of complex interventions to improve health. *British Medical Journal* 2000;321:694–6.

7   Gilbody S, Bower P, Fletcher J, Richards D, Sutton A. Collaborative care for depression: a systematic review and cumulative meta-analysis. *Archives of Internal Medicine* 2006;166:2314–21.

8   Bijl D, van Marwijk W, de Haan M, van Tilburg W, Beekman A. Effectiveness of disease management programmes for recognition, diagnosis and treatment of depression in primary care: a review. *European Journal of General Practice* 2004;10:6–12.

9   Gensichen J, Beyer M, Muth C, Gerlach F, Von Korff M, Ormel J. Case management to improve major depression in primary health care: a systematic review. *Psychological Medicine* 2005;35:1–8.

10 Lehman A. A review of instruments for measuring quality of life outcomes in mental health. In: N Miller, K Magruder, editors. *Cost-effectiveness of Psychotherapy: A Guide for Practitioners, Researchers and Policy Makers*. New York: Oxford University Press, 1999;174–81.

11 Mintz J, Bond G, Mintz L. Assessing work function in mental health research. In: N Miller, K Magruder, editors. *Cost-effectiveness of Psychotherapy: A Guide for Practitioners, Researchers and Policy Makers*. New York: Oxford University Press, 1999;194–205.

12 Kaplan R. Health-related quality of life in mental health services evaluation. In: N Miller, K Magruder, editors. *Cost-effectiveness of Psychotherapy: A Guide for Practitioners, Researchers and Policy Makers*. New York: Oxford University Press, 1999:160–73.

13 Barkham M, Evans C, Margison F *et al*. The rationale for developing and implementing core outcome batteries for routine use in service settings and psychotherapy outcome research. *Journal of Mental Health* 1999;7:35–47.

14 Higgins J, Green S. *Cochrane Handbook for Systematic Reviews of Interventions Version 5.0.1*. In: Cochrane Collaboration, 2009. Available at: www.cochrane-handbook.org

15 Gilbody S, Whitty P, Grimshaw J, Thomas R. Educational and organisational interventions to improve the management of depression in primary care: a systematic review. *Journal of the American Medical Association* 2003;289:3145–51.

16 Egger M, Juni P, Bartlett C, Holenstein F, Sterne J. How important are comprehensive literature searches and the assessment of trial quality in systematic reviews? Empirical study. *Health Technology Assessment* 2003;7:1–76.

17 Moher D, Liberati A, Tetzlaff J, Altman D, PRISMA group. Preferred reporting items for systematic reviews and meta-analyses: the PRISMA statement. *British Medical Journal* 2009;339:b2535.

18 Simpson S, Corney R, Fitzgerald P, Beecham J. A randomised controlled trial to evaluate the effectiveness and cost-effectiveness of counselling patients with chronic depression. *Health Technology Assessment* 2000;4:1–83.

19 Schulz K, Grimes D. Allocation concealment in randomised trials: defending against deciphering. *Lancet* 2002;359:614–18.

20 Schulz K, Chalmers I, Hayes R, Altman D. Empirical evidence of bias: dimensions of methodological quality associated with estimates of treatment effects in controlled trials. *Journal of the American Medical Association* 1995;273:408–12.

21 Wood L, Egger M, Gluud L *et al.* Empirical evidence of bias in treatment effect estimates in controlled trials with different interventions and outcomes: meta-epidemiological study. *British Medical Journal* 2008;336:601–5.

22 Lipsey M, Wilson D. *Practical Meta-Analysis*. Newbury Park, CA: Sage, 2001.

23 Sutton A, Abrams K, Jones D, Sheldon T, Song F. Systematic reviews of trials and other studies. *Health Technology Assessment* 1998;2:1–272.

5

Education and training

Simon Gilbody

Case study

Dr Stevens is aware that guidelines have recently been issued on the management of depression by the government and professional organizations. Her managers are very keen to ensure that local practice is informed by the latest evidence and have printed several hundred copies of the summary sheet (outlining the main guideline recommendations) and also arranged for an external trainer to come and give a seminar at a local educational event.

Dr Stevens looks at the summary guideline and puts it on the pile of 15 other things she needs to read that day, and also wonders whether someone from the practice ought to go to the event. She is sure that the guidelines are sensible and a useful summary of the best available evidence. However, she wonders generally about whether guidelines actually make a difference to patient care. She also wonders whether educational events are worth the effort, since there are other calls on her time and other means of keeping her practice up to date. She wonders what the evidence shows in this respect.

Education and training (through the production and dissemination of guidelines and the provision of educational events) are commonly used means of improving the quality of patient care. Guidelines are frequently produced as part of national quality improvement efforts, and depression is no exception. If effective, education and training represents the optimal method of improving the quality of care in terms of efficiency, since the practice of a large number of primary care professionals can be altered through passive dissemination of educational materials or short training courses.

In depression, there is a long history of the employment of education and training, based on the results of an important education and training study conducted on the Swedish island of Gotland in the 1980s.[1,2] Within this study, an education and training intervention was associated with an apparent reduction in suicide

Depression in Primary Care: Evidence and Practice, ed. Simon Gilbody and Peter Bower. Published by Cambridge University Press. © Cambridge University Press 2011.

rates and an increase in antidepressant prescription. However, the Gotland study employed a weak methodological design (an 'interrupted time series'),[3] with no comparable control group, which makes it vulnerable to confounding and low internal validity. Far more robust designs have been subsequently employed in the evaluation of education and training, and all randomized controlled trial evidence is considered in this chapter.

Inclusion criteria

Studies included in the review were randomized controlled trials of education and training, involving guidelines or educational events. For guidelines, we adopted the Institute of Medicine's definition of a 'systematically developed statement to assist practitioner and patient decisions about appropriate health care for specific clinical circumstances'.[4] Educational events were defined as one or more events where primary care professionals were given information about depression by an expert in the condition. The content of educational events could vary, from didactic sessions through to those requiring active participation, homework or the use of recognized educational strategies such as 'role play'.

Results

We found 10 randomized trials examining the impact of educational and training studies (Table 5.1).[5–15] Four were conducted in the UK,[6,8,9,11] four in the USA[5,7,10,14] and one each in the Netherlands[12] and Canada.[13] Only seven reporting data on patient depression outcomes and are included in the analysis. Patients included in the studies were identified through a variety of screening questionnaires and diagnostic systems.

All guideline-based studies included an evidence-supported guideline but with a variable level of educational support. There was significant variation in the content and process of the educational intervention to support the guideline; ranging from a single three-hour group-based event,[7] through to more intensive series of educational events with significant role play among participants.[9] Some studies had detailed one-to-one input from a content expert through *academic detailing*[14] (i.e. face-to-face education of professionals) or the use of decision support systems to provide patient-specific guideline reminders following an educational intervention.[10] The largest study was based in the UK, and used a multifaceted educational intervention targeted at all members of the primary care team, based on established educational principles (see Chapter 2, Box 2.2 for a more detailed description of this study).[11]

The quality data extracted from the studies are shown in Table 5.1. Studies ranged from 'low' to 'medium' quality and often had high levels of patient attrition.

Seven studies of eight different interventions measured patient-level outcomes of depression and were included in the meta-analysis.[6,7,9–11,13,14] Only one study

Table 5.1 Education and training model versus usual primary care for depression – studies included in the review

Study reference(s) Study population	Educational intervention	Sample size	Allocation concealment	Attrition	Quality
Baker et al., 2001[6] UK Primary care professionals and patients with depression identified by their primary care professional	Primary care professionals provided with guidelines on the management of depression in primary care and an interview conducted to identify barriers to implementation, with feedback Control group had guidelines issued with no implementation analysis	64 primary care professionals 402 patients	Not clear	44% (intervention) 45% (control)	Low
Brown et al., 2000[7] USA Primary care professionals and patients with probable depression	Continuous quality improvement Educational visits to each primary care professional on guideline-based recognition and management of depression with handouts System supports given (such as access to depression questionnaires and telephone access to a psychiatrist)	160 primary care professionals 928 patients	Not clear	24% (overall)	Low
Gask et al., 2004[9] UK Primary care professionals and patients with depression defined by Hamilton Depression Scale	10-hour multifaceted intervention directed at senior GPs Educational strategy – training GPs in skills for the assessment and management of depression	38 primary care professionals 395 patients	Randomization by practice according to computer-generated random number tables	36% (intervention) 39% (control)	Medium

Table 5.1 (*cont.*)

Study reference(s) Study population	Educational intervention	Sample size	Allocation concealment	Attrition	Quality
Goldberg et al., 1998[14] USA Primary care professionals and patients with and without depression	Academic detailing – physician opinion leader paid a 15-minute visit and gave 'detailing sheets' mimicking pharmaceutical advertisements Continuous quality improvement plus academic detailing Distribution of educational materials, educational meetings, audit and feedback, local consensus processes	95 primary care professionals 4051 patients (with or without depression), and 2154 (with physician-recognized depression)	Not clear	Not clear	Low
Rollman et al., 2002[10] USA Primary care professionals from academically affiliated practices and patients with DSM Major Depressive Disorder	'Active care' electronic reminder of depression diagnosis and patient-specific recommendations (based on guidelines) given to clinician during the clinical encounter 'Passive care' paper-based reminder of diagnosis of depression, with no patient-specific treatment recommendations	15 primary care professionals 212 patients	Not clear	13% (intervention 1), 9% (intervention 2), 13% (control)	Medium
Thompson et al., 2000[11] UK Primary care practices and patients assessed as depressed on the Hospital Anxiety and Depression Scale	Educational materials, meetings and outreach	59 practices 1247 patients with depression	Practices randomly assigned by computer	48% (intervention) 46% (control)	Medium

Worrall et al., 1999[13] Canada Primary care profes- sionals and patients with depression diagnosed by Centre for Epidemiological Studies Depression Scale	Case-based educational strategy on improved recognition and management of depression in line with Canadian guidelines	42 primary care professionals 147 patients	Assigned by random number tables	Not clear	Medium

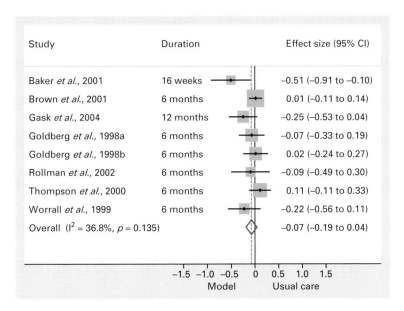

Study	Duration	Effect size (95% CI)
Baker *et al.*, 2001	16 weeks	−0.51 (−0.91 to −0.10)
Brown *et al.*, 2001	6 months	0.01 (−0.11 to 0.14)
Gask *et al.*, 2004	12 months	−0.25 (−0.53 to 0.04)
Goldberg *et al.*, 1998a	6 months	−0.07 (−0.33 to 0.19)
Goldberg *et al.*, 1998b	6 months	0.02 (−0.24 to 0.27)
Rollman *et al.*, 2002	6 months	−0.09 (−0.49 to 0.30)
Thompson *et al.*, 2000	6 months	0.11 (−0.11 to 0.33)
Worrall *et al.*, 1999	6 months	−0.22 (−0.56 to 0.11)
Overall ($I^2 = 36.8\%$, $p = 0.135$)		−0.07 (−0.19 to 0.04)

Figure 5.1 Effectiveness of educational and training model in the short term.

		Incremental effectiveness		
		−	0	+
Incremental costs	+		Kendrick *et al.*, 2001;[15] Gask *et al.*, 2004[9]	
	0			
	−			

Figure 5.2 Education and training model – permutation matrix for costs and effects.

reported effects over the long-term, and all studies were thus combined in a single analysis. The pooled analysis found no significant effect (effect size 0.07, 95% CI −0.19 to 0.04, $I^2 = 37\%$, Figure 5.1). Two studies reported cost and effectiveness, and the results were in the 'higher cost-equivalent effectiveness' quadrant.[9,15] The permutation plot is shown in Figure 5.2.

REFERENCES

1 Rutz W, von Knorring L, Walinder J. Frequency of suicide on Gotland after systematic postgraduate education for general practitioners. *Acta Psychiatrica Scandinavica* 1989;80:151–4.

2 Rutz W, von Knorring L, Walinder J. Long-term effects of an educational program for general practitioners given by the Swedish Committee for the prevention and treatment of depression. *Acta Psychiatrica Scandinavica* 1992;85:83–8.

3 Gilbody S, Whitty P. Improving the delivery and organisation of mental health services: beyond the conventional randomised controlled trial. *British Journal of Psychiatry* 2002;180:13–18.

4 Institute of Medicine. *Guidelines for Clinical Practice: From Development to Use.* Washington, DC: National Academy Press, 1992.

5 Andersen S, Harthorn B. Changing the psychiatric knowledge of primary care physicians: the effects of a brief intervention on clinical diagnosis and treatment. *General Hospital Psychiatry* 1990;12:177–90.

6 Baker R, Reddish S, Robertson N, Hearnshaw H, Jones B. Randomised controlled trial of tailored strategies to implement guidelines for the management of patients with depression in general practice. *British Journal of General Practice* 2001;51:737–41.

7 Brown J, Shye D, McFarland B, Nichols G, Mullooly J, Johnson R. Controlled trial of CQI and academic detailing to implement a clinical practice guideline for depression. *Joint Commission Journal on Quality Improvement* 2001;26:39–54.

8 Freemantle N, Nazareth I, Eccles M, Wood J, Haines A, the Evidence-based OutReach (EBOR) trialists. A randomised controlled trial of the effect of educational outreach by community pharmacists on prescribing in UK general practice. *British Journal of General Practice* 2002;52:290–5.

9 Gask L, Dowrick C, Dixon C *et al.* A pragmatic cluster randomized controlled trial of an educational intervention for GPs in the assessment and management of depression. *Psychological Medicine* 2004;34:63–72.

10 Rollman B, Hanusa B, Lowe H, Gilbert T, Kapoor W, Schulberg H. A randomized trial using computerized decision support to improve treatment of major depression in primary care. *Journal of General Internal Medicine* 2002;17:493–503.

11 Thompson C, Kinmonth A, Stevens L *et al.* Effects of a clinical practice guideline and practice-based education on detection and outcome of depression in primary care: Hampshire Depression Project randomised controlled trial. *Lancet* 2000;355:185–91.

12 van Eijk M, Avorn J, Porsius A, de Boer A. Reducing prescribing of highly anticholinergic antidepressants for elderly people: randomised trial of group versus individual academic detailing. *British Medical Journal* 2001;322:1–6.

13 Worrall G, Angel J, Chaulk P, Clarke C, Robbins M. Effectiveness of an educational strategy to improve family physicians' detection and management of depression: a randomized controlled trial. *Canadian Medical Association Journal* 1999;161:37–40.

14 Goldberg H, Wagner E, Fihn S *et al.* A randomized controlled trial of CQI teams and academic detailing: can they alter compliance with guidelines? *Joint Commission Journal on Quality Improvement* 1998;24:130–42.

15 Kendrick T, Stevens L, Bryant A *et al.* Hampshire Depression Project: changes in the process of care and cost consequences. *British Journal of General Practice* 2001;51:911–13.

6

Consultation-liaison

John Cape, Craig Whittington and Peter Bower

Case study

Dr Stevens has been approached by the local organization responsible for mental health in the community. The team that provides care for patients in her practice has offered to come to meet all the primary care professionals in its area to discuss 'better ways of working with primary care'. The possibility of a specialist holding a clinic in the practice once per month has been suggested. At the moment, when Dr Stevens wants the expert opinion of someone in the community team, she has to make a written referral, and it takes several weeks for patients to be seen for a routine assessment.

Many written referrals are sent back (with the patient not having been seen) if they do not have a disorder of sufficient severity or do not meet the criteria that have been set down by the team. The team is very busy and seems to focus most of its efforts on people with disorders such as schizophrenia, although this has never been officially stated.

Dr Stevens does not necessarily want all the patients with depression in the practice to be seen by a psychiatrist, psychologist or other specialist. She realizes that this is not the best use of their time or expertise. However, she would like the opportunity to discuss more complex cases and to receive some advice about management and referral. There is no facility for this to happen at present. She enjoys the challenge of mental health and thinks she could learn something from working more closely with the specialists in the mental health team.

The meeting is due to happen next week, and Dr Stevens is quite keen to receive the input of a specialist in the practice on a regular basis. She wonders whether there is any research to support this approach and has heard about the concept of 'consultation-liaison', although she has seen this happen only when she used to work in the local general hospital.

Depression in Primary Care: Evidence and Practice, ed. Simon Gilbody and Peter Bower. Published by Cambridge University Press. © Cambridge University Press 2011.

The consultation-liaison model involves specialists (such as psychiatrists) entering into an ongoing educational relationship with the primary care team, in order to support them in caring for depressed patients who are currently undergoing care (see Chapter 2). Consultation-liaison could potentially represent the optimal trade-off between effectiveness and efficiency, because the bulk of treatment is delivered by primary care staff (thus maximizing access, equity and reducing costs), but the benefits of specialist expertise are available to deal with difficult cases and improve effectiveness in those cases where routine primary care may not be sufficient.

Inclusion criteria

Studies included in the review were randomized controlled trials of consultation-liaison interventions for depressed patients in primary care. As noted earlier, the definition of consultation-liaison varies according to context, and some collaborative care interventions include aspects of consultation-liaison as part of the complex intervention.

Consultation-liaison was defined as an intervention where patients were seen by a mental health professional for a maximum of one or two sessions. The purpose of these sessions was restricted to assessment and advice to the primary care professional about management, but in the majority of cases no treatment was provided by the mental health professional.

Results

Five studies of consultation-liaison were identified.[1–5] The studies were conducted in the USA,[2,3] UK,[5] Italy[1] and Taiwan.[4]

Patients included in three studies had depressive disorders or high levels of depressive symptoms,[1,2,5] while one study recruited patients with 'common mental health disorders'[4] and one recruited distressed patients with high levels of utilization of health services in the previous 12 months.[3] Patients were recruited by screening in four of five studies [1–3,5] and by referral from general medical clinics in one study.[4]

There was significant variation in the content and process of the consultation-liaison intervention. In a study of depressed high utilizers of care in the USA, patients had an interview with a psychiatrist followed by a second joint interview with the psychiatrist and primary care professional. This led to the negotiation of a treatment plan. Primary care professionals also received written feedback on their patient and a follow-up conference with the psychiatrist to review progress.[3] In the study in Italy, the psychiatrist provided an assessment, met with primary care professionals in case review meetings and used those meetings to discuss management strategies. Each patient was discussed at three meetings.[1] In a study in elderly depressed patients in the UK, a member of a community mental health team

Table 6.1 Consultation-liaison model versus usual primary care for depression – studies included in the review

Study reference Patient population	Consultation-liaison format	Specialist	Sample size	Allocation concealment	Attrition	Quality
Arthur et al., 2002[5] UK Patients identified as depressed recruited via health check by practice nurses	Mental health assessment and written report to the GP, with a proportion followed up by a community mental health team for further treatment	Member of the community mental health team	93	Sealed, opaque, numbered envelopes	32% (intervention), 15% (control)	Medium
Berti Ceroni et al., 2002[1] Italy Patients with depressive disorders (major depressive disorder, minor depression, sub-syndromal depression) recruited via screening	Assessment of patient, with assessment fed back to primary care practitioner that the patient met 'caseness' criteria, followed by meetings with the primary care practitioners for case review and discussion of management strategies. Each intervention patient was discussed on three separate occasions	Psychiatrist	92	Not clear	13% at one year	Medium
Dobscha et al., 2006[2] USA Patients with depression recruited from telephone screening	A single telephone call from a depression care manager providing education and support, followed by feedback on treatment recommendations to the primary care practitioner after weekly review of medication, appointment and outcome data.	Depression care manager and psychiatrist	375	Not clear	14% (intervention), 18% (control) at 6 months	Medium

Table 6.1 (*cont.*)

Study reference Patient population	Consultation-liaison format	Specialist	Sample size	Allocation concealment	Attrition	Quality
	Where patients did not adequately improve, a consultation appointment with the psychiatrist was arranged, with the option for referral ongoing speciality mental healthcare					
Katon et al., 1992[3] USA High-utilizing patients screening high on symptom checklist	Interview with psychiatrist followed by second joint interview with psychiatrist and primary care practitioner and patient to negotiate treatment plan. The primary care practitioner also received written feedback and a treatment protocol for the patient from the psychiatrist plus one later follow-up conference with the psychiatrist to review each patient	Psychiatrist	251	Not clear	3% (intervention), 4% (control) at 6 months	Medium
Liu et al., 2007[4] Taiwan Patients with common mental disorders recruited from general medical clinics in a general hospital	Consultation from a psychiatrist, making recommendations for management to the treating general medical physician, with follow-up meetings with the patient if the psychiatrist believed that it was indicated	Psychiatrist	254 (148 between consultation-liaison and usual care)	Not clear	9% (intervention), 22% (control)	Medium

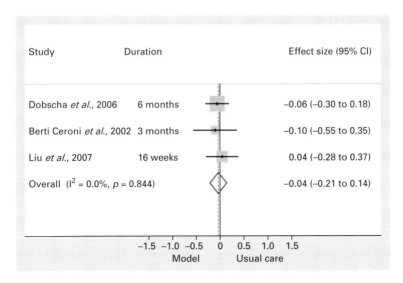

Figure 6.1 Effectiveness of the consultation-liaison model in the short term.

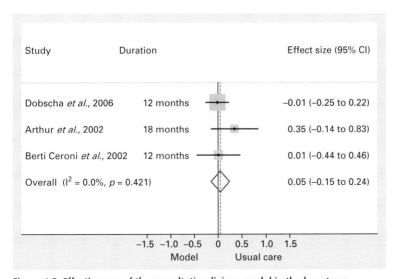

Figure 6.2 Effectiveness of the consultation-liaison model in the long term.

assessed the patient and provided a written report to the primary care professional. The assessment involved data on mental health history and use of medication. A minority of patients were also followed up by the mental health professional, but only after formal agreement with the primary care professional.[5] In the Taiwanese study of patients with common mental disorders, the psychiatrist met with the patient and provided recommendations for management, with a minority of patients receiving follow-up meetings with the psychiatrist.[4] Finally, the study in depressed patients in the USA used consultation from a depression care manager (similar to a case manager as defined in collaborative care models – see Chapter 7). However, the intervention was more limited in scope than collaborative care, with a focus on education, exploring barriers to treatment and adherence, and encouraging communication with the primary care professional. A 'decision support team' (comprising care managers and psychiatrists) then provided quarterly feedback to the primary care professional following review of medication and appointment data. If patients failed to benefit, a consultation appointment with the psychiatrist could be arranged, or the decision support team might arrange referral for specialist mental health support.[2]

The quality data extracted from the studies are shown in Table 6.1. Using the criteria outlined in Chapter 3, all studies were considered 'medium' quality.

Three studies[1,2,4] provided data for meta-analysis of depression outcomes in the short-term, and found no significant effect (effect size –0.04, 95% CI –0.21 to 0.14, $I^2 = 0$, Figure 6.1).

Three studies[1,2,5] provided data for meta-analysis of depression outcomes in the long-term, and found no significant effect (effect size 0.05, 95% CI –0.15 to 0.24, $I^2 = 0$, Figure 6.2).

No studies reported cost-effectiveness outcomes.

REFERENCES

1 Berti Ceroni G, Rucci P, Beradi D, Ceroni F, Katon W. Case review vs. usual care in primary care patients with depression: a pilot study. *General Hospital Psychiatry* 2002;24:71–80.

2 Dobscha S, Corson K, Hickman D, Perrin N, Kraemer D, Gerrity M. Depression decision support in primary care: a cluster randomized trial. *Annals of Internal Medicine* 2006;145:477–87.

3 Katon W, Von Korff M, Lin E *et al.* A randomized trial of psychiatric consultation with distressed high utilisers. *General Hospital Psychiatry* 1992;14:86–9.

4 Liu S, Huang H, Yeh Z *et al.* Controlled trial of problem-solving therapy and consultation-liaison for common mental disorders in general medical settings in Taiwan. *General Hospital Psychiatry* 2007;29:402–8.

5 Arthur A, Jagger C, Lindesay J, Matthews R. Evaluating a mental health assessment for older people with depressive symptoms in general practice: a randomised controlled trial. *British Journal of General Practice* 2002;52:202–7.

7

Collaborative care

Simon Gilbody

Case study

Dr Stevens has many patients with depression and she notes that several of them do not take medication that she believes might help, or do not return for their follow-up appointments. She would like more of her patients to receive psychological interventions (such as cognitive-behavioural therapy), but the waiting lists are quite long.

Money has become available to employ a 'graduate worker' in her practice to help with problems such as depression. The 'graduate worker' is a relatively junior professional with a psychology background, who has been on a training course to provide skills in some aspects of depression care, including simple psychological treatments. She wonders what care these workers might offer, and remembers reading about enhancements of care developed in the USA that apply the principles of 'chronic disease management'. She has already found these sorts of enhancements helpful for patients with other long-term conditions such as diabetes and arthritis.

She does a quick online search and finds some resources detailing various interventions described as 'collaborative care', 'case management' and 'enhanced care'. There are many trials and several meta-analyses of these interventions and she downloads copies of these.

This seems positive and helpful, but she will need to convince her partners and the manager of the local mental health services that the 'graduate worker' should be employed to help deliver 'collaborative care', rather than other forms of mental healthcare.

The collaborative care model involves treating depression through the combined efforts of a primary care professional, a specialist mental health professional and a case manager, with the care coordinated by the case manager to ensure optimum symptom management and follow-up.[1] Case managers provide care face-to-face or

Depression in Primary Care: Evidence and Practice, ed. Simon Gilbody and Peter Bower. Published by Cambridge University Press. © Cambridge University Press 2011.

over the telephone and have access to specialist support from the specialist mental health professional (such as a psychiatrist or psychologist). Case management often includes both helping patients with antidepressant medication (working in collaboration with the primary care professional) and brief psychological therapy (often a 'minimal' psychological intervention – see Chapters 8 and 11).

Collaborative care builds on the notion of depression as a chronic disease[2] (see Chapter 1) and seeks to enhance the care for people with depression through a range of strategies (see Chapter 2), all provided in a structured and systematic way.[1,3] This model of care originated in the USA within managed care services and it is unsurprising that the majority of studies have been conducted in this setting. However, a number of studies have now been conducted in other settings, including European countries[4] and less-well-resourced non-European healthcare systems.[5]

Inclusion criteria

We included randomized controlled trials of patients with depression being managed in primary care settings using a collaborative care approach. For the purposes of the review, collaborative care was broadly defined as a multifaceted intervention that involved combinations of three distinct professionals (a case manager, a primary care practitioner and a mental health specialist)[6] working in collaboration on a treatment plan, through agreed protocols, proactive follow-up and structured liaison and feedback.

Results

We found 43 comparisons of collaborative care and a usual-care condition (see Table 7.1).[4,5,7–44] All but 11 were conducted in the USA.[7,12–14,16–29,32,34–43]

Patients included those with major depression according to a diagnostic standard and those identified on the basis of significant depression symptoms. Some trials were restricted to certain types of patients (such as females or the elderly) and some were restricted to patients who had recently begun antidepressant treatment. The collaborative care interventions were very varied. Case managers included a range of professionals, such as graduate psychologists, mental health nurses, social workers and pharmacists (see Table 7.1).

Twenty-three studies were rated as 'high' quality,[4,5,9,15,23–29,31,33–35,37,38,40–42] 13 as 'medium' quality[7,11,14,16–18,21,22,30,32,36,39,44] and 7 as 'low' quality.[8,10,12,13,19,20,43] (see Table 7.1).

In the analysis of short-term outcomes, collaborative care was associated with a 'small' but significant improvement in depression symptoms (effect size = –0.28, 95% CI –0.32 to –0.23, I^2 = 48%, Figure 7.1).

Table 7.1 Collaborative care model versus usual primary care for depression – studies included in the review

Study reference(s) Patient population	Collaborative care intervention	Sample size	Allocation concealment	Attrition	Quality
Adler et al., 2004[7] USA Adults with DSM IV major depression or dysthymia	Pharmacist working with primary care professionals to meet medication guidelines	533	'Computerised coin flip' Concealment not clear	13%	Medium
Akerblad et al., 2003[8] Sweden Adults with major depression and an indication for antidepressants	Case management and medication monitoring by a GP	1031	Randomization and concealment not clear	Unclear	Low
Araya et al., 2003[5] Chile Female adults with major depression	Collaborative care (including psycho-education) by a non-medical health worker	240	Computer-generated random number tables, with concealment	12%	High
Blanchard et al., 1995[10] UK Elderly patients with depression warranting clinical intervention	Case management by community nurse supported by multidisciplinary team	96	Not clear	33%	Low
Bosmans et al., 2006[9] Netherlands Elderly patients with DSM IV major depressive disorder not already in receipt of antidepressants	Disease management by a general practitioner	125	Computer-generated random number tables Concealment not clear	14%	High
Brook 2003 et al., [11,45] Netherlands Adults with depressive complaints, prescribed new antidepressant	Case management and coaching by community pharmacists	147	Randomized by computer and sealed envelopes	27%	Medium

Table 7.1 (*cont.*)

Study reference(s) Patient population	Collaborative care intervention	Sample size	Allocation concealment	Attrition	Quality
Bruce et al., 2004[12] USA Elderly people with major depression, dysthymia and minor depression	Collaborative care through case managers (social workers, nurses and psychologists)	598	Cluster randomization by practice Practices matched into pairs and allocated by flipping coin	23%	Low
Callahan et al., 1994[13] USA Elderly patients with newly diagnosed depression	Screening and case management by physician	175	Random number tables	Unclear	Low
Capoccia et al., 2004[14] USA Adults with depression, prescribed a new antidepressant	Collaborative care through pharmacist medication monitoring	74	Not clear	5%	Medium
Chew-Graham et al., 2007[15] UK Elderly depressed patients	Case management by a community psychiatric nurse (including self-help) and liaison with primary care and old-age psychiatry	105	Computerized randomization with minimization	8%	High
Coleman et al., 1999[16] USA Frail elderly	Chronic care clinics from physician, nurse and pharmacist	169	Randomization by practice using 'simple randomization'	11%	Medium
Datto et al., 2003[17] USA Adults with depressive symptoms	Telephone disease management by a nurse	61	Randomization by practice Method not clear	18%	Medium

Study	Intervention	n	Randomization		
Dietrich et al., 2004[18] USA Adults with major depression and dysthymia (DSM IV), starting or changing treatment	Collaborative care through case managers, supported by psychiatrists	405	Practices randomized in pairs by the flip of a coin	20%	Medium
Ell et al., 2007[19] USA Elderly patients in receipt of home nursing	Training of home health nurses and clinical depression specialists in collaborative care, including problem solving	311	Methods of randomization not clear	44%	Low
Finley et al., 1999[20] USA Adults with current major depression, prescribed a new antidepressant	Pharmacist medication management and follow-up	125	Not clear	33%	Low
Fortney et al., 2007[21] USA Patients with depression	Collaborative care with telemedicine support	395	Not clear	9%	Medium
Hunkeler et al., 2000[22] USA Adults with major depression or dysthymia, prescribed a new antidepressant	Collaborative care through nurse telephone support	302	Not clear	15%	Medium
Jarjoura et al., 2004[23] USA Adults with major depression not currently in treatment	Collaborative care through guidelines for primary care professionals and nurse behavioral care	121	Randomized with sealed envelopes	10%	High
Katon et al., 1995[24] USA Adults with depression prescribed a new antidepressant	Collaborative care from psychiatrist and medication monitoring	217	Computer generated	15%	High

Table 7.1 (*cont.*)

Study reference(s) Patient population	Collaborative care intervention	Sample size	Allocation concealment	Attrition	Quality
Katon et al., 1996[25] USA Adults with depression prescribed a new antidepressant	Collaborative care with behavioural treatment and medication monitoring	153	Computer generated	16%	High
Katon et al., 1999[26] USA Adults at high risk of persistent depression, recurrent depression or dysthymia	Collaborative care by a psychiatrist	228	Randomization by computer, with stratification	16%	High
Katon et al., 2001[27] USA Adults, prescribed a new antidepressant, at high risk of relapse	Collaborative care relapse prevention programme	386	Computer generated	10%	High
Katon et al., 2004[28] USA Adults with diabetes and depressive symptoms	Collaborative care for depression through clinical nurse specialist	329	Computer generated	12%	High
Katzelnick et al., 2000[29] USA Adult high utilizers of services, with depressive symptoms	Collaborative care depression management programme through treatment coordinators	407	Computer generated	6%	High
Mann et al., 1998[31] UK Adults with depression	Case management and medication monitoring by nurses	419	Sealed envelope opened only at the end of first assessment interview	9%	High

Study	Intervention	N	Randomization method	%	Quality
McMahon et al., 2007[30] UK Adults with depression who had failed to respond to antidepressants	Case management delivered by primary care mental health workers	62	Randomization codes generated by a researcher and held at a separate site	42%	Medium
Oslin et al., 2003[32] USA Adults with depression or dysthymia, at-risk drinking	Telephone disease management by a behavioural health specialist	97	Randomization by physician – method not specified; concealment not clear	23%	Medium
Peveler et al., 1999[33] UK Patients with diagnosis of depression, prescribed a new antidepressant	Nurse delivered antidepressant counselling	160	Randomization by computer with sealed envelopes to maintain concealment	11%	High
Richards et al., 2008[4] UK Depressed patients	Collaborative care by nurse, counsellor and occupational therapist, and graduate mental health workers	117	Randomization by computer at remote site	16%	High
Rickles et al., 2005[34] USA Adults with depression, prescribed a new antidepressant	Medication monitoring by a pharmacist	63	Random selection from sealed envelopes	5%	High
Rost et al., 2001a[35] USA Adults with major depression, prescribed a new antidepressant, recently treated	Primary care team training in collaborative care and enhanced depression treatment	243	Randomization of practices in blocks	10%	High
Rost 2001b[35] USA Adults with major depression, prescribed a new antidepressant, beginning new episode	Primary care team training in collaborative care and enhanced depression treatment	189	Randomization of practices in blocks	10%	High

Table 7.1 (*cont.*)

Study reference(s) Patient population	Collaborative care intervention	Sample size	Allocation concealment	Attrition	Quality
Rubenstein et al., 2006[36] USA Patients with major depression	Quality improvement intervention including clinician education and case management	567	Randomization of practices by computer	23%	Medium
Simon et al., 2000[37] USA Adults with depression, prescribed a new antidepressant	Feedback and telephone case management	392	Computer-generated random numbers	5%	High
Simon et al., 2004a[38] USA Adults with depression, prescribed a new antidepressant	Collaborative care through telephone care management	402	Computer-generated random numbers without blocking or stratification	11%	High
Simon et al., 2004b[38] USA Adults with depression, prescribed a new antidepressant	Collaborative care through telephone care management and psychotherapy	393	Computer-generated random numbers without blocking or stratification	11%	High
Swindle et al., 2003[39] USA Adults with major depression, dysthymia or partially remitted major depression	Case management by clinical nurse specialists	268	Coin toss, concealment not clear	17%	Medium
Unützer et al., 2003[40] USA Elderly with major depression, dysthymia or both	Collaborative care (including problem solving) by a care manager	1801	Randomization by computer at coordinating centre	17%	High

Study	Intervention	N	Randomization		
Wang et al., 2007[41] USA Working age adults with depression	Telephone care management	604	Randomization by computerized procedure	9%	High
Wells et al., 2000a[42] USA Adults with major depression or dysthymia	Depression quality improvement through nurse medication management	867	Randomization of clinicians with identification of patients prior to knowledge of allocation status	15%	High
Wells et al., 2000b[42] USA Adults with major depression or dysthymia	Depression quality improvement through facilitated access to psychological therapy	932	Randomization of clinicians with identification of patients prior to knowledge of allocation status	15%	High
Whooley et al., 2000[43] USA Elderly with depressive symptoms	Case finding and educational groups run by a psychiatric nurse	331	Not clear	38%	Low
Wilkinson et al., 1993[44] UK Patients with depressive disorders judged as needing antidepressants	Medication management by a nurse	61	Randomization information included in sealed pre-packed protocols; concealment not clear	5%	Medium

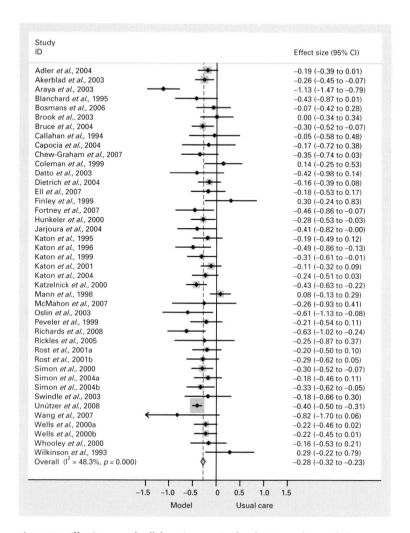

Figure 7.1 Effectiveness of collaborative care in the short term (6 months).

In the analysis of longer-term outcomes, collaborative care was associated with a small but generally significant improvement in depression symptoms (effect size at 12 months –0.43, 95% CI –0.50 to –0.37, I^2 = 89%; effect size at 18 months –0.32, 95% CI –0.39 to –0.25, I^2 = 84%; effect size at 24 months –0.24, 95%CI –0.30 to –0.17, I^2 = 81%; effect size at 60 months –0.15, 95%CI –0.30 to –0.00, I^2 = 0; Figure 7.2).

Ten studies reported cost-effectiveness outcomes,[24–27,29,35,41,42,46,47] and the results were concentrated in the 'higher cost–higher effectiveness' quadrant. The permutation plot is shown in Figure 7.3.

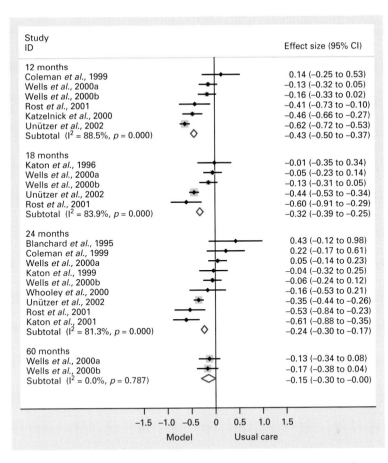

Study ID		Effect size (95% CI)
12 months		
Coleman et al., 1999		0.14 (−0.25 to 0.53)
Wells et al., 2000a		−0.13 (−0.32 to 0.05)
Wells et al., 2000b		−0.16 (−0.33 to 0.02)
Rost et al., 2001		−0.41 (−0.73 to −0.10)
Katzelnick et al., 2000		−0.46 (−0.66 to −0.27)
Unützer et al., 2002		−0.62 (−0.72 to −0.53)
Subtotal (I² = 88.5%, p = 0.000)		−0.43 (−0.50 to −0.37)
18 months		
Katon et al., 1996		−0.01 (−0.35 to 0.34)
Wells et al., 2000a		−0.05 (−0.23 to 0.14)
Wells et al., 2000b		−0.13 (−0.31 to 0.05)
Unützer et al., 2002		−0.44 (−0.53 to −0.34)
Rost et al., 2001		−0.60 (−0.91 to −0.29)
Subtotal (I² = 83.9%, p = 0.000)		−0.32 (−0.39 to −0.25)
24 months		
Blanchard et al., 1995		0.43 (−0.12 to 0.98)
Coleman et al., 1999		0.22 (−0.17 to 0.61)
Wells et al., 2000a		0.05 (−0.14 to 0.23)
Katon et al., 1999		−0.04 (−0.32 to 0.25)
Wells et al., 2000b		−0.06 (−0.24 to 0.12)
Whooley et al., 2000		−0.16 (−0.53 to 0.21)
Unützer et al., 2002		−0.35 (−0.44 to −0.26)
Rost et al., 2001		−0.53 (−0.84 to −0.23)
Katon et al., 2001		−0.61 (−0.88 to −0.35)
Subtotal (I² = 81.3%, p = 0.000)		−0.24 (−0.30 to −0.17)
60 months		
Wells et al., 2000a		−0.13 (−0.34 to 0.08)
Wells et al., 2000b		−0.17 (−0.38 to 0.04)
Subtotal (I² = 0.0%, p = 0.787)		−0.15 (−0.30 to −0.00)

−1.5 −1.0 −0.5 0 0.5 1.0 1.5

Model   Usual care

Figure 7.2 Effectiveness of collaborative care in the medium and long term (12–60 months).

		Incremental effectiveness		
		−	0	+
Incremental costs	+			Katon et al., 1995[24,28]; 1996[25,48]; 1999[26,49,50]; Katzelnick et al., 2000[29,52]; Simon et al., 2000[46]; Wells et al., 2000[42,54]; Katon et al., 2001[27,51]; Rost et al., 2001[35,53]; Hedrick et al., 2003[47,55]; Wang et al., 2007[41]
	0			Katon et al., 1999[26,50]
	−			

Figure 7.3 Collaborative care model – permutation matrix for costs and effects.

REFERENCES

1 Von Korff M, Goldberg D. Improving outcomes of depression: the whole process of care needs to be enhanced. *British Medical Journal* 2001;323:948–9.

2 Wagner EH, Austin BT, Von Korff M. Organizing care for patients with chronic illness. *Milbank Journal Quarterly* 1996;74:511–44.

3 Von Korff M, Glasgow RE, Sharpe M. ABC of psychological medicine: Organising care for chronic illness. *British Medical Journal* 2002;325:92–4.

4 Richards DA, Lovell K, Gilbody S *et al.* Collaborative care for depression in UK primary care: a randomized controlled trial. *Psychological Medicine* 2008;38:279–87.

5 Araya R, Rojas G, Fritsch R *et al.* Treating depression in primary care in low income women in Santiago, Chile: a randomised controlled trial. *Lancet* 2003;361:995–1000.

6 Katon W, Von Korff M, Lin E, Simon GE. Rethinking practitioner roles in chronic illness: the specialist primary care physician and the practice nurse. *General Hospital Psychiatry* 2001;23:138–44.

7 Adler DA, Bungay KM, Wilson IB *et al.* The impact of a pharmacist intervention on 6-month outcomes in depressed primary care patients. *General Hospital Psychiatry* 2004;26:199–209.

8 Akerblad AC, Bengtsson F, Ekselius L, von Knorring L. Effects of an educational compliance enhancement programme and therapeutic drug monitoring on treatment adherence in depressed patients managed by general practitioners. *International Clinical Psychopharmacology* 2003;18:347–54.

9 Bosmans J, de Bruijne M, van Hout H *et al.* Cost-effectiveness of a disease management program for major depression in elderly primary care patients. *Journal of General Internal Medicine* 2006;21:1020–6.

10 Blanchard MR, Waterreus A, Mann AH. The effect of primary care nurse intervention upon older people screened as depressed. *International Journal of Geriatric Psychiatry* 1995;10:289–98.

11 Brook O, Van Hout B, Nieuwenhuyse H. Effects of coaching by community pharmacists on psychological symptoms of antidepressant users: a randomised controlled trial. *European Neuropsychopharmacology* 2003;13:347–54.

12 Bruce M, Ten Have T, Reynolds C *et al.* Reducing suicidal ideation and depressive symptoms in depressed older primary care patients. *Journal of the American Medical Association* 2004;291:1081–91.

13 Callahan C, Hendrie H, Dittus R, Brater D, Hui S, Tierney W. Improving treatment of late life depression in primary care: a randomized clinical trial. *Journal of the American Geriatrics Society* 1994;42:839–46.

14 Capoccia K, Boudreau D, Blough D *et al.* Randomized trial of pharmacist interventions to improve depression care and outcomes in primary care. *American Journal of Health System Pharmacy* 2004;61:364–72.

15 Chew-Graham CA, Lovell K, Roberts C *et al.* A randomised controlled trial to test the feasibility of a collaborative care model for the management of depression in older people. *British Journal of General Practice* 2007;57:364.

16 Coleman EA, Grothaus LC, Sandhu N, Wagner EH. Chronic care clinics: a randomized controlled trial of a new model of primary care for frail older adults. *Journal of the American Geriatrics Society* 1999;47:775–83.

17 Datto CJ, Thompson R, Horowitz D, Disbot M, Oslin DW. The pilot study of a telephone disease management program for depression. *General Hospital Psychiatry* 2003;25:169–77.

18 Dietrich AJ, Oxman TE, Williams JW, Jr. *et al.* Going to scale: re-engineering systems for primary care treatment of depression. *Annals of Family Medicine* 2004;2:301–4.

19 Ell K, Unützer J, Aranda M, Gibbs NE, Lee PJ, Xie B. Managing depression in home health care: a randomized clinical trial. *Home Health Care Services Quarterly* 2007;26:81–104.

20 Finley P, Rens H, Gess S, Loiue C. Case management of depression by clinical pharmacists in a primary care setting. *Formulary* 1999;34:864–70.

21 Fortney JC, Pyne JM, Edlund MJ *et al.* A randomized trial of telemedicine-based collaborative care for depression. *Journal of General Internal Medicine* 2007;22:1086–93.

22 Hunkeler EM, Meresman JF, Hargreaves WA *et al.* Efficacy of nurse telehealth care and peer support in augmenting treatment of depression in primary care. *Archives of Family Medicine* 2000;9:700–8.

23 Jarjoura D, Polen A, Baum E, Kropp D, Hetrick S, Rutecki G. Effectiveness of screening and treatment for depression in ambulatory indigent patients. *Journal of General Internal Medicine* 2004;19:78–84.

24 Katon W, Von Korff M, Lin E *et al.* Collaborative management to achieve treatment guidelines. Impact on depression in primary care. *Journal of the American Medical Association* 1995;273:1026–31.

25 Katon W, Robinson P, Von Korff M *et al.* A multifaceted intervention to improve treatment of depression in primary care. *Archives of General Psychiatry* 1996;53:924–32.

26 Katon W, Von Korff M, Lin E *et al.* Stepped collaborative care for primary care patients with persistent symptoms of depression: a randomized trial. *Archives of General Psychiatry* 1999;56:1109–15.

27 Katon W, Rutter C, Ludman EJ *et al.* A randomized trial of relapse prevention of depression in primary care. *Archives of General Psychiatry* 2001;58:241–7.

28 Katon WJ, Von Korff M, Lin EHB *et al.* The Pathways Study: A randomized trial of collaborative care in patients with diabetes and depression. *Archives of General Psychiatry* 2004;61:1042–9.

29 Katzelnick DJ, Simon GE, Pearson SD *et al.* Randomized trial of a depression management program in high utilizers of medical care. *Archives of Family Medicine* 2000;9:345–51.

30 McMahon L, Foran KM, Forrest SD *et al.* Graduate mental health worker case management of depression in UK primary care: a pilot study. *British Journal of General Practice* 2007;57:880.

31 Mann A, Blizard R, Murray J. An evaluation of practice nurses working with general practitioners to treat people with depression. *British Journal of General Practice* 1998;48:875–9.

32 Oslin D, Sayers S, Ross J *et al.* Disease management for depression and at risk drinking via telephone in an older population of veterans. *Psychosomatic Medicine* 2003;65:931–7.

33 Peveler R, George C, Kinmonth AL, Campbell M, Thompson C. Effect of antidepressant drug counselling and information leaflets on adherence to drug treatment in primary care: randomised controlled trial. *British Medical Journal* 1999;319:612–15.

34 Rickles N, Svarstad BL, Statz-Paynter JL, Taylor LV, Kobak KA. Pharmacist telemonitoring of antidepressant use: effects on pharmacist-patient collaboration. *Journal of the American Pharmaceutical Association* 2005;45:344–53.

35 Rost K, Nutting PA, Smith J, Werner J, Duan N. Improving depression outcomes in community primary care practice: a randomised trial of the QuEST intervention. *Journal of General Internal Medicine* 2001;16:143–9.

36 Rubenstein LV, Meredith LS, Parker LE *et al.* Impacts of evidence-based quality improvement on depression in primary care: a randomized experiment. *Journal of General Internal Medicine* 2006;21:1027.

37 Simon G, Von Korff M, Rutter C, Wagner E. Randomised trial of monitoring, feedback and management of care by telephone to improve treatment of depression in primary care. *British Medical Journal* 2000;320:550–4.

38 Simon GE, Ludman EJ, Tutty S, Operskalski B, Korff MV. Telephone psychotherapy and telephone care management for primary care patients starting antidepressant treatment: a randomized controlled trial. *Journal of the American Medical Association* 2004;292:935–42.

39 Swindle R, Rao J, Helmy A *et al.* Integrating clinical nurse specialists into the treatment of primary care patients with depression. *International Journal of Psychiatry in Medicine* 2003;33:17–37.

40 Unützer J, Katon W, Callahan CM *et al.* Collaborative care management of late-life depression in the primary care setting: a randomized controlled trial. *Journal of the American Medical Association* 2003;288:2836–45.

41 Wang PS, Simon GE, Avorn J *et al.* Telephone screening, outreach, and care management for depressed workers and impact on clinical and work productivity outcomes: a randomized controlled trial. *Journal of the American Medical Association* 2007;298:1401–11.

42 Wells KA, Sherbourne C, Schoenbaum M *et al.* Impact of disseminating quality improvement programmes for depression in managed primary care: a randomized controlled trial. *Journal of the American Medical Association* 2000;283:212–20.

43 Whooley MA, Stone B, Soghikian K. Randomized trial of case-finding for depression in elderly primary care patients. *Journal of General Internal Medicine* 2000;15:293–300.

44 Wilkinson G, Allen P, Marshall E. The role of the practice nurse in the management of depression in general practice: treatment adherence to antidepressant medication. *Psychological Medicine* 1993;23:229–37.

45 Brook O, van Hout H, Nieuwenhuyse H, Heerdink E. Impact of coaching by community pharmacists on drug attitude of depressive primary care patients and acceptability to patients; a randomized controlled trial. *European Neuropsychopharmacology* 2003;13:1–9.

46 Simon GE, VonKorff M, Rutter C, Wagner E. Randomised trial of monitoring, feedback, and management of care by telephone to improve treatment of depression in primary care. *British Medical Journal* 2000;320:550–4.

47 Hedrick SC, Chaney EF, Felker B *et al.* Effectiveness of collaborative care depression treatment in Veterans' Affairs primary care. *Journal of General Internal Medicine* 2003;18:9–16.

48 Von Korff M, Katon W, Bush T *et al.* Treatment costs, cost offset, and cost-effectiveness of collaborative management of depression. *Psychosomatic Medicine* 1998;60:143–9.

49 Lin EH, VonKorff M, Russo J *et al.* Can depression treatment in primary care reduce disability? A stepped care approach. *Archives of Family Medicine* 2000;9:1052–8.

50 Simon GE, Katon WJ, VonKorff M *et al.* Cost-effectiveness of a collaborative care program for primary care patients with persistent depression. *American Journal of Psychiatry* 2001;158:1638–44.

51 Simon GE, Von Korff M, Ludman EJ *et al.* Cost-effectiveness of a program to prevent depression relapse in primary care. *Medical Care* 2002;40:941–50.

52 Simon GE, Manning WG, Katzelnick DJ *et al.* Cost-effectiveness of systematic depression treatment for high utilizers of general medical care. *Archives of General Psychiatry* 2001;58:181–7.

53 Pyne JM, Rost KM, Zhang M, Williams DK, Smith J, Fortney J. Cost-effectiveness of a primary care depression intervention. *Journal of General Internal Medicine* 2003;18:432–41.

54 Schoenbaum M, Unützer J, Sherbourne C *et al.* Cost-effectiveness of practice-initiated quality improvement for depression: results of a randomized controlled trial. *Journal of the American Medical Association A* 2001;286:1325–30.

55 Liu CF, Hedrick SC, Chaney EF *et al.* Cost-effectiveness of collaborative care for depression in a primary care veteran population. *Psychiatric Services* 2003;54:698–704.

8

Referral

Peter Bower

Case study

The local healthcare organization that is responsible for Dr Stevens has been talking
for some time about the lack of access to psychological therapies for patients with
depression. A recent national initiative has been launched to increase the provision
of psychological therapies, and the organization has applied for funds to be part of
this initiative. However, there is a lack of clarity about how they should go about
this, and a poor understanding of 'who does what' in psychological therapies.

For some time Dr Stevens' practice has employed a counsellor. Patients seem
to like this, and Dr Stevens and her partners value ready access to someone who
offers this sort of support. However, she isn't sure whether counselling is the best or
most effective form of psychological therapy for disorders such as depression. She
knows a little about cognitive-behavioural therapy and this is available from local
psychologists, but there are very long waiting times for this service.

Her primary care colleagues are keen on the idea of greater access to psychological therapy in their practice. Dr Stevens wonders whether they should just buy in
the services of another counsellor, or introduce other treatments.

She wonders what the evidence is to support various types of psychological therapy for depression.

The referral model most frequently involves the provision of psychological therapies
in primary care (see Chapter 2). There are a variety of relevant psychological therapies
available, and major debates about their relative effectiveness and cost effectiveness,
which have been a feature of the field for many years[1,2] and continue to this day.[3,4]

In the UK and elsewhere, evidence about the effectiveness of psychological
therapies is dominated by cognitive-behavioural therapy (CBT). This structured
treatment is informed by the theories of Beck and others,[5] and incorporates both
cognitive and behavioural elements. Patients are taught to challenge negative
thinking, monitor their behaviour and undertake homework tasks. The treatment
is generally structured and time limited and is amenable to description and standardization through use of a treatment manual.[6]

Depression in Primary Care: Evidence and Practice, ed. Simon Gilbody and Peter Bower. Published by
Cambridge University Press. © Cambridge University Press 2011.

There are many other varieties of psychological therapy that have been provided in primary care, such as problem solving,[7] counselling,[8] psychodynamic therapy[9] and interpersonal therapy,[10] as well as treatments that combine psychological therapy with a more educational focus (so-called *psycho-education*).[11] For the purposes of the current book, CBT will be used as the exemplar for the referral model, although the comparative clinical and cost effectiveness of alternative psychological therapies will also be considered.

Inclusion criteria

Studies included in the review were randomized controlled trials of CBT delivered by a therapist working in a referral model, to patients with depressive disorder or depressive symptoms in the primary care setting. Where CBT was delivered as part of other interventions (e.g. GP training, collaborative care), these studies were included in their relevant chapters.

Results

Six studies were identified (Table 8.1).[8,12–19] All but one were conducted in the UK. Patients included those with major depression according to a diagnostic standard[14,15,16,18] and those identified on the basis of significant depression symptoms.[8,19] Therapists were mainly psychologists[8,14,15,18,19] but also included social workers.[16] In one case, therapists had received additional training from a specialist CBT centre.[18] The CBT interventions ranged in length from 6 to 12 sessions[8,14] to up to 20 sessions plus additional 'booster' sessions.[18] Individual session length ranged from 30 minutes[15] to 60 minutes.[18]

One study was considered 'high' quality,[8] one 'medium' quality[14] and four 'low' quality.[15,16,18,19]

In the analysis of short-term outcomes, the referral model was associated with a moderate but significant improvement in depression symptoms (effect size –0.38, 95% CI –0.63 to –0.13, $I^2 = 0\%$, Figure 8.1).

In the analysis of long-term outcomes, the referral model was associated with a small and non-significant improvement in depression symptoms (effect size –0.17, 95% CI to –0.52 to 0.18, $I^2 = 0\%$, Figure 8.2).

Only one study reported cost-effectiveness outcomes, and the results were in the 'equivalent cost–equivalent effectiveness' quadrant in the long term. The permutation plot is shown in Figure 8.3.

Other interventions in referral models

As noted above, CBT delivered in a conventional format through a series of 50–60 minute meetings with a therapist is only one exemplar of a referral model, and there are a number of alternative interventions and ways of delivering the treatment.

Table 8.1 Referral model versus usual primary care for depression – studies included in the review

Study reference Patient population	Therapy format	Therapist(s)	Sample size	Allocation concealment	Attrition	Quality
King 2000[8,12,13] UK Patients with depression and mixed anxiety and depression	6–12 50-minute sessions.	11 psychologists	134	Sealed opaque envelopes	4m (91%) 12m (83%)	High
Scott and Freeman 1992[14] UK Patients with depression	10 50-minute appointments	2 senior research clinical psychologists	121	Sealed envelopes	4w (93%) 16w (93%)	Medium
Scott et al., 1997[15] UK Patients with major depressive disorder	6 30-minute sessions	Therapist with post-graduate qualification in cognitive therapy	48	Not clear	7w (71%) 19w (56%) 32w (54%) 58w (50%)	Low
Ross 1985[16,17] UK Patients with major depressive disorder	12 45-minute sessions for individual treatment 12 90-minute sessions for group treatment	Social worker	67	Not clear	Not clear Not clear Not clear	Low
Teasdale et al., 1984[18] UK Patients with major depressive disorder	Up to 20 1-hour sessions, plus 2 booster sessions.	2 experienced clinical psychologists trained by Centre for Cognitive Therapy in Philadelphia	44	Not clear	Post 3m (77%)	Low
Bolton 2001[19] Australia Patients with depression	8–10 sessions of 50 minutes.	Registered psychologist	17	Not clear	10w (94%)	Medium

w, weeks; m, months.

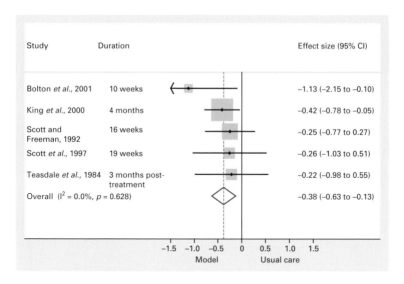

Figure 8.1 **Effectiveness of the referral model in the short term.**

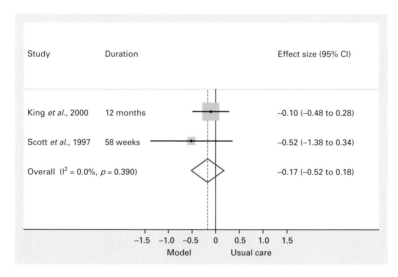

Figure 8.2 **Effectiveness of the referral model in the long term.**

		Incremental effectiveness		
		–	0	+
	+			
Incremental costs	0		King 2000[8,12,13]	
	–			

Figure 8.3 **Referral model – permutation matrix for costs and effects.**

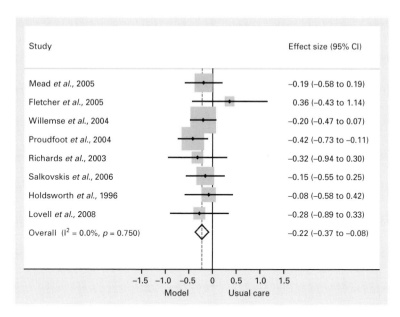

Study		Effect size (95% CI)
Mead *et al.*, 2005		−0.19 (−0.58 to 0.19)
Fletcher *et al.*, 2005		0.36 (−0.43 to 1.14)
Willemse *et al.*, 2004		−0.20 (−0.47 to 0.07)
Proudfoot *et al.*, 2004		−0.42 (−0.73 to −0.11)
Richards *et al.*, 2003		−0.32 (−0.94 to 0.30)
Salkovskis *et al.*, 2006		−0.15 (−0.55 to 0.25)
Holdsworth *et al.*, 1996		−0.08 (−0.58 to 0.42)
Lovell *et al.*, 2008		−0.28 (−0.89 to 0.33)
Overall (I^2 = 0.0%, p = 0.750)		−0.22 (−0.37 to −0.08)

−1.5 −1.0 −0.5   0   0.5   1.0 1.5
Model   Usual care

Figure 8.4 Effectiveness of minimal interventions in the referral model in the short term.

The comparative clinical effectiveness of different psychological therapies delivered within this model has been the subject of much debate. Previous systematic reviews of treatments such as counselling have suggested broadly similar patterns of results to those presented here, i.e. a modest but significant benefit in the short term, which may not endure in the longer term.[20] Other meta-analyses that have examined a range of psychological therapies generally report similar findings in terms of clinical effectiveness in the short and long term, although the precise estimates vary according to the studies included in the review.[21] Meta-analyses that have compared different types of therapy (such as CBT, problem solving and counselling) have reported some variation in the effectiveness of treatments. For example, a recent meta-analysis reported effect sizes of 0.42 for CBT, 0.19 for problem solving and 0.27 for other therapies.[22] Although such differences are of interest, the magnitude of the differences is relatively small, and the limited number of available studies and the possibility of other confounding variables means that such differences must be interpreted with caution. Direct comparisons of different therapies in primary care are rare, but one study which did assess CBT and counselling together in a randomized controlled trial found little difference in terms of clinical or cost effectiveness.[8,12,13] At present, the conservative conclusion may be that these treatments are of broadly similar effectiveness, at least when delivered in primary care.

Although CBT is often viewed as a treatment of choice, it is potentially expensive and resource limitations mean that it is then difficult to access in a timely fashion. However, many elements of CBT can be provided in forms that do not require face-to-face access to a therapist (indeed, work outside the psychological therapy session as 'homework' is a major part of the treatment). There is a great deal of interest in alternative ways of delivering CBT that do not require such large amounts of face-to-face contact with a therapist. These are often known as 'minimal' or 'self-help' interventions, and involve CBT techniques delivered via written materials, computers, the Internet and other media.[23] Such treatments may be as effective as traditional therapist-delivered forms of CBT, but require a fraction of the therapist's time, thus improving efficiency and access.

These interventions and the technologies to deliver them are relatively new and the evidence base is developing rapidly, although many of the early trials were conducted outside primary care.[24–26] Although we did not subject these trials to the same systematic assessment as the core models, Figure 8.4 shows the results of a number of trials of these technologies. Although there are examples of highly effective interventions,[27,28] the evidence base in primary care suggests that the overall clinical effectiveness of these interventions is 'small' (effect size −0.22, 95% CI −0.37 to −0.08, $I^2 = 0\%$)[27–35] and their promise in terms of cost effectiveness remains to be proved.

REFERENCES

1 Smith M, Glass G, Miller T. *The Benefits of Psychotherapy*. Baltimore, MD: Johns Hopkins University Press, 1980.
2 Eysenck H. The effects of psychotherapy: an evaluation. *Journal of Consulting and Clinical Psychology* 1952;16:319–24.
3 Tarrier N. Commentary: Yes, cognitive-behaviour therapy may well be all you need. *British Medical Journal* 2002;324:291–2.
4 Holmes J. All you need is cognitive-behaviour therapy. *British Medical Journal* 2002;324:288–90.
5 Beck A, Rush A, Shaw B, Emery G. *Cognitive Therapy of Depression*. New York: Guilford Press, 1979.
6 Churchill R, Hunot V, Corney R et al. A systematic review of controlled trials of the effectiveness and cost-effectiveness of brief psychological treatments for depression. *Health Technology Assessment* 2001;5:1–173.
7 Mynors-Wallis L, Gath D, Day A, Baker F. Randomised controlled trial of problem solving treatment, antidepressant medication, and combined treatment for major depression in primary care. *British Medical Journal* 2000;320:26–30.
8 Ward E, King M, Lloyd M et al. Randomised controlled trial of non-directive counselling, cognitive-behaviour therapy and usual GP care for patients with depression. I: Clinical effectiveness. *British Medical Journal* 2000;321:1383–8.
9 Brodaty H, Andrews G. Brief psychotherapy in family practice – a controlled prospective intervention trial. *British Journal of Psychiatry* 1983;143:11–19.
10 Schulberg H, Block M, Madonia M et al. Treating major depression in primary care practice: eight month clinical outcomes. *Archives of General Psychiatry* 1996;53:913–19.
11 Brown J, Cochrane R, Hancox T. Large scale health promotion stress workshops for the general public: a controlled evaluation. *Behavioural and Cognitive Psychotherapy* 2000;28:139–51.
12 King M, Sibbald B, Ward E et al. Randomised controlled trial of non-directive counselling, cognitive-behaviour therapy and usual general practitioner care in the management

of depression as well as mixed anxiety and depression in primary care. *Health Technology Assessment* 2000;4:1–83.

13 Bower P, Byford S, Sibbald B *et al*. Randomised controlled trial of non-directive counselling, cognitive-behaviour therapy and usual GP care for patients with depression. II: Cost effectiveness. *British Medical Journal* 2000;321:1389–92.

14 Scott A, Freeman C. Edinburgh primary care depression study: treatment outcome, patient satisfaction, and cost after 16 weeks. *British Medical Journal* 1992;304:883–7.

15 Scott C, Tacchi M, Jones R, Scott J. Acute and one-year outcome of a randomised controlled trial of brief cognitive therapy for major depressive disorder in primary care. *British Journal of Psychiatry* 1997;171:131–4.

16 Ross M, Scott M. An evaluation of the effectiveness of individual and group cognitive therapy in the treatment of depressed patients in an inner city health centre. *Journal of the Royal College of General Practitioners* 1985;35:239–42.

17 Scott M, Stradling S. Group cognitive therapy for depression produces clinically significant reliable change in community-based settings. *Behavioural Psychotherapy* 1990;18:1–19.

18 Teasdale J, Fennel M, Hibbert G, Amies P. Cognitive therapy for major depressive disorder in primary care. *British Journal of Psychiatry* 1984;144:400–6.

19 Bolton P, Fergusson K, Parker S, Orman J. Randomised controlled trial of cognitive-behavioural therapy and routine GP care for major depression. *Medical Journal of Australia* 2001;175:118–19.

20 Bower P, Rowland N. Effectiveness and cost effectiveness of counselling in primary care. *Cochrane Database of Systematic Reviews* 2006;Issue 3. Art. No.: CD001025. DOI: 10.1002/14651858.CD001025.pub2.

21 Bortolotti B, Menchetti M, Bellini F, Montaguti M, Berardi D. Psychological interventions for major depression in primary care: a meta analytic review of randomized controlled trials. *General Hospital Psychiatry* 2008;30:293–302.

22 Cuijpers P, Van Straten A, van Schaik A, Andersson G. Psychological treatment of depression in primary care: a meta-analysis. *British Journal of General Practice* 2009;59:51–60.

23 Newman M, Erickson T, Przeworski A, Dzus E. Self-help and minimal-contact therapies for anxiety disorders: is human contact necessary for therapeutic efficacy? *Journal of Clinical Psychology* 2003;59:251–74.

24 Gellatly J, Bower P, Hennessey S, Richards D, Gilbody S, Lovell K. What makes self-help interventions effective in the management of depressive symptoms? Meta-analysis and meta-regression. *Psychological Medicine* 2007;37:1217–28.

25 Anderson L, Lewis G, Araya R *et al*. Self-help books for depression: how can practitioners and patients make the right choice? *British Journal of General Practice* 2005;55:387–92.

26 Den Boer P, Wiersma D, Van Den Bosch R. Why is self-help neglected in the treatment of emotional disorders? A meta-analysis. *Psychological Medicine* 2004;34:959–71.

27 Proudfoot J, Ryden C, Everitt B *et al*. Clinical efficacy of computerised cognitive-behavioural therapy for anxiety and depression in primary care: randomised controlled trial. *British Journal of Psychiatry* 2004;185:46–54.

28 Proudfoot J, Goldberg D, Mann A, Everitt B, Marks I, Gray J. Computerized, interactive, multimedia cognitive-behavioural program for anxiety and depression in general practice. *Psychological Medicine* 2003;33:217–27.

29 Fletcher J, Lovell K, Bower P, Campbell M, Dickens C. Process and outcome of a non-facilitated self-help manual for anxiety and depression in primary care: a pilot study. *Behavioral and Cognitive Psychotherapy* 2005;33:319–31.

30 Holdsworth N, Paxton R, Seidel S, Thomson D, Shrubb S. Parallel evaluations of new guidance materials for anxiety and depression in primary care. *Journal of Mental Health* 1996;5:195–207.

31 Mead N, MacDonald W, Bower P, Lovell K, Richards D, Bucknall A. The clinical effectiveness of guided self-help versus waiting list control in the management of anxiety and depression: a randomised controlled trial. *Psychological Medicine* 2005;35:1633–43.

32 Richards A, Barkham M, Cahill J, Richards D, Williams C, Heywood P. PHASE: a randomised, controlled trial of supervised self-help cognitive behavioural therapy in primary care. *British Journal of General Practice* 2003;53:764–70.

33 Salkovskis P, Rimes K, Stephenson D, Sacks G, Scott J. A randomized controlled trial of the use of self-help materials in addition to standard general practice treatment of depression compared to standard treatment alone. *Psychological Medicine* 2006;36:325–33.

34 Willemse G, Smit F, Cuijpers P, Tiemens B. Minimal contact psychotherapy for sub-threshold depression in primary care: randomised trial. *British Journal of Psychiatry* 2004;185:416–21.

35 Lovell K, Bower P, Richards D *et al*. Developing guided self-help for depression using the Medical Research Council complex interventions framework: a description of the modelling phase and results of an exploratory randomised controlled trial. *BMC Psychiatry* 2008;8:91.

9

Summary of the evidence

Peter Bower and Simon Gilbody

The purpose of this book was to outline the application of the techniques of evidence-based practice and systematic review to decisions about the best way to manage depression in primary care.

After discussing the philosophy and techniques of evidence-based practice, Chapters 5, 6, 7 and 8 provided a detailed assessment of the evidence concerning each model. Figure 9.1 shows the evidence concerning the short-term effectiveness of each model placed on a single graph, for comparison (the restriction to the short-term data reflecting that this represents the bulk of the available evidence).

A variety of schemes are available to make sense of the evidence identified by a systematic review. One important issue is the magnitude of the effect suggested by the review. Individual studies used a variety of measures of treatment effect, but the process of meta-analysis standardizes the measure of effect across studies to make them comparable, and then provides a pooled assessment of the evidence, summarizing the effect of a number of studies.

The evidence reviews in Chapters 5, 6, 7 and 8 report this summary effect size. There are a number of interpretations of that measure, some of which were outlined in Box 3.1. The most popular is the simple scheme popularized by Cohen, whereby the pooled effect size is characterized as 'small' (effect size around 0.2), 'moderate' (effect size around 0.5) and 'large' (effect size around 0.8).[1] Although these categories are fairly arbitrary, there is some evidence that they reflect meaningful groupings.[2,3]

When outcomes are dichotomous (i.e. patients are 'depressed' or 'not depressed' for example), estimates of the effects of treatment are often provided in terms of what is called *number need to treat* (NNT). This is a useful index, because it tells the health professional how many patients need to be treated with a certain intervention (i.e. referred to a collaborative care intervention) to avoid one additional negative outcome (i.e. a patient remaining 'depressed' six months later). The NNT is often used to interpret the effects of medical interventions. Effect sizes such as those calculated in this book can be translated to an approximate NNT (if one

Depression in Primary Care: Evidence and Practice, ed. Simon Gilbody and Peter Bower. Published by Cambridge University Press. © Cambridge University Press 2011.

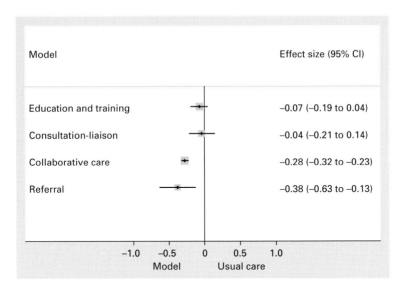

Figure 9.1 Overall summary of the short-term effectiveness evidence.

accepts certain assumptions).[4] An effect size of 0.2 approximates to an NNT of around 9, 0.3 to around 6, and 0.4 to around 5.

A complication relates to the comparison of the effects sizes between models. Whereas the comparisons between intervention and control groups in a single trial are based on randomization, the same is not true of the comparisons between models. So it is legitimate to conclude that there is no evidence that consultation-liaison is better than usual care in improving depression symptoms. However, it is not strictly legitimate to conclude that the effectiveness of the referral model is higher than that of collaborative care. Although the estimate is higher (0.38 vs. 0.27), we do not know whether comparing those estimates is legitimate, because there may be other differences between the studies that might account for those differences. Although there are some advanced statistical techniques that can be used to explore these issues through what is called 'indirect comparisons',[5] the most rigorous method would be to design and conduct a randomized controlled trial directly comparing the effectiveness of the collaborative care and referral models, to see whether the differences found in the reviews endure in a direct randomized comparison. Some of the models have already been compared in this way. Hedrick and colleagues explored the relative effectiveness of collaborative care and consultation-liaison models in the treatment of depressed patients, and found that collaborative care resulted in more rapid improvements in depression.[6]

The amount of available evidence about cost effectiveness was very limited. The importance of formal cost-effectiveness analyses has only been acknowledged in depression care relatively recently, and most of the available studies relate to collaborative care. The most consistent finding is that collaborative care is associated with increases in costs as well as effectiveness, and the little evidence that exists for

> **Box 9.1** GRADE: Quality of evidence and definitions[7]
>
> - High quality – Further research is very unlikely to change our confidence in the estimate of effect
> - Moderate quality – Further research is likely to have an important impact on our confidence in the estimate of effect and may change the estimate
> - Low quality – Further research is very likely to have an important impact on our confidence in the estimate of effect and is likely to change the estimate
> - Very low quality – Any estimate of effect is very uncertain

the referral model also suggests that this is the case. At present, the evidence on cost effectiveness is not a strong basis for favouring one model over another.

Chapter 2 also identified other dimensions that are relevant when considering the performance of a model. The impact of a model on access to care is important, given what is known about the low levels of treatment among depressed patients in the community. However, the randomized controlled trials identified in the reviews are not effective at testing the impact on access. What is required is a study that measures the impact of a model of care on access to care among a defined population of patients, and such assessments are rare. The benefits of different models on this dimension are therefore not well understood, although it is likely that the increased costs associated with the collaborative care and referral models means that their advantages in terms of access may be limited. The limitations of the evidence base in terms of assessments of access are also relevant for assessments of equity, which would require knowledge of the impact of the model on access among different patient populations.

Finally, there is the issue of the patient-centredness of care. Many of the trials in the reviews include some data on patient satisfaction, but the measurements of patient-satisfaction and patient-centredness are at an early stage, and the measurements that are available are generally not comparable across studies. The increasing importance placed on this dimension means that effective measurement will be a priority in the future, and such measurements may provide another way of distinguishing between models.

Grading the evidence

Guideline developers have described different ways of grading evidence to provide clear advice to professionals and patients. This involves an assessment of both the *quality of the evidence* (see Box 9.1) and a statement about the *strengths of recommendations* that result from the evidence review (Box 9.2).

Assessments of quality relate to the likelihood that further research will change confidence in the results. If there is a significant amount of evidence, low heterogeneity in the estimates of effectiveness, and the precision of the estimate is high, then further research is unlikely to impact on our confidence. If limited evidence

Box 9.2 Factors that affect the strength of a recommendation[7]

Factor	Examples of strong recommendations	Examples of weak recommendations
Quality of evidence	Randomized trials and other well-designed studies	Studies with low internal validity such as before and after studies without control groups
Uncertainty about the balance between desirable and undesirable effects	Clear evidence of benefit with minimal side effects	Small clinical benefits with significant side effects or high prevalence of adverse outcomes in some patients
Uncertainty or variability in values and preferences	Clear evidence on effects on quality of life and function	Uncertain value placed on outcomes such as symptom relief
Uncertainty about whether the intervention represents a wise use of resources	Evidence of benefit associated with low cost or cost offset	Evidence of benefit associated with high costs and resource use

exists, the effects among studies are highly variable or the precision is low, then the results may be highly sensitive to the publication of new data.

Finally, quality of evidence about outcomes cannot be the sole decision-making criterion. Box 9.2 highlights other factors that might be taken into account in terms of the strengths of recommendations, because high-quality evidence does not necessarily imply strong recommendations, and strong recommendations can arise from low-quality evidence. This is because it is necessary to take into account whether the desirable effects of an intervention clearly outweigh the undesirable effects (whether those undesirable effects relate to side effects, adverse outcomes or increased costs). If the benefits outweigh those undesirable effects, guidelines can offer strong recommendations. On the other hand, when the trade-offs are less certain, weaker recommendations are necessary.

The most important in the present context may be the issues of patient-centredness. Providing care in line with the preferences of patients is a key outcome for health services (see Chapter 2), and there is some evidence that patients value certain aspects of mental health treatment delivery more than others. For example, psychological therapy is highly valued,[8] whereas many patients are more ambivalent about the benefits of medication.[9,10] Guideline development panels are constantly grappling with the problems of making conventional systematic reviews sensitive to this sort of patient experience data, although at present the data are used more to provide context for the review rather than being explicitly integrated into the evidence synthesis. Integrating quantitative and qualitative data is a major area of research interest, but the challenges are significant.[11-13] Some of the principles of systematic review can be applied to the synthesis of qualitative data.[14]

At present, the evidence for collaborative care meets the criteria for high quality, given the amount of evidence and the precision with which the effect is known. However, it could be argued that the estimate of the effectiveness of the treatment is small, and thus a strong recommendation might be inappropriate. The more limited evidence bases for the other models are best characterized as being between moderate- and low-quality assessments, and in all cases further research is required to increase the precision of the estimates and the confidence with which they can be used to make policy and clinical decisions. This means that in all cases, only weak recommendations could be made.

It may strike some as surprising that a comprehensive assessment of scientific evidence through systematic review involves such subjective and qualitative judgements when final decisions are made. Partly this reflects limitations in terms of the overall amount of evidence, and partly a lack of agreed and coherent systems for comparing and weighing different types of evidence (such as effectiveness, cost and patient-centredness). Although evidence-based practice seeks to systematize the decision-making process as far as possible and maximize the use of scientific evidence, it is difficult to see that it could or should ever make the decision-making process entirely mechanistic.

REFERENCES

1 Cohen J. *Statistical Power Analysis for the Behavioural Sciences (2nd edition)*. New Jersey: Lawrence Erlbaum, 1988.

2 Lipsey M. *Design Sensitivity: Statistical Power for Experimental Research*. Newbury Park, CA: Sage, 1990.

3 Lipsey M, Wilson D. The efficacy of psychological, educational and behavioural treatment. *American Psychologist* 1993;48:1181–209.

4 Kraemer H, Kupfer D. Size of treatment effects and their importance to clinical research and practice. *Biological Psychiatry* 2006;59:990–6.

5 Song F, Altman D, Glenny A, Deeks J. Validity of indirect comparison for estimating efficacy of competing interventions: empirical evidence from published meta-analyses. *British Medical Journal* 2003;326:472

6 Hedrick S, Chaney E, Felker B *et al*. Effectiveness of collaborative care depression treatment in Veterans' Affairs Primary Care. *Journal of General Internal Medicine* 2003;18:9–16.

7 Guyatt G, Oxman A, Vist E *et al*. GRADE: an emerging consensus on rating quality of evidence and strength of recommendations. *British Medical Journal* 2008;336:924–6.

8 Priest R, Vize C, Roberts A, Roberts M, Tylee A. Lay people's attitudes to treatment of depression: results of opinion poll for Defeat Depression Campaign just before its launch. *British Medical Journal* 1996;313:858–9.

9 Knudsen P, Hansen E, Traulsen J, Eskildsen K. Changes in self-concept while using SSRI antidepressants. *Qualitative Health Research* 2002;12:932–44.

10 Grime J, Pollock K. Information versus experience: a comparison of an information leaflet on antidepressants with lay experience of treatment. *Patient Education and Counseling* 2004;54:361–8.

11 Dixon-Woods M, Agarwal S, Jones D, Young B, Sutton A. Synthesising qualitative and quantitative evidence: a review of possible methods. *Journal of Health Services Research and Policy* 2005;10:45–53.

12 Dixon-Woods M, Bonas S, Booth A *et al.* How can systematic reviews incorporate qualitative research? A critical perspective. *Qualitative Research* 2006;6:27–44.

13 Thomas J, Harden A, Oakley A *et al.* Integrating qualitative research with trials in systematic reviews. *British Medical Journal* 2004;328:1010–12.

14 Khan N, Bower P, Rogers A. Guided self-help in primary care mental health: a meta synthesis of qualitative studies of patient experience. *British Journal of Psychiatry* 2007;191:206–11.

10

Making it happen

Peter Bower and Simon Gilbody

Previous chapters have outlined the evidence base concerning different models of depression care in primary care. The reviews of research have identified the relative weight of evidence for each model in terms of clinical and cost-effectiveness, and the data were summarized in Chapter 9. The next step is therefore translating that evidence into routine clinical practice. However, as highlighted by the Institute of Medicine, 'between the health care we have and the care we could have lies not just a gap but a chasm'.[1]

The chasm between research and practice remains one of the most important limitations to evidence-based practice. Despite advances in scientific methods and the ease of accessing evidence, using evidence to change clinical practice remains a significant challenge.[2] A classic example outside of depression is the use of streptokinase in heart attacks. Figure 10.1 shows a 'cumulative' meta-analysis, where the results of randomized trials are ordered by date, and the plot shows the accumulation of evidence over time, with the gradual increase in the precision of the estimate (shown by the narrowing confidence intervals around the estimate) as more studies were completed. The scientific evidence that streptokinase was effective was sufficiently strong by the early 1970s, but the treatment did not become routine until 1986. There are few clearer demonstrations of the problems of the research–practice 'chasm'.

There is a similar example in depression care. Figure 10.2 shows the cumulative meta-analysis plot for the collaborative care model outlined in Chapter 7. The plot would suggest that sufficient evidence was available concerning the effectiveness of collaborative care in 2000, at least in terms of the evidence being sufficiently precise to give high confidence that the treatment was superior to usual care (notwithstanding arguments about the size of the effect). However, the use of collaborative care in practice is still relatively limited even today.

Why is there such a gap between research and clinical practice? Understanding that gap first requires an understanding of the relationship between research and clinical practice. The development of evidence-based practice has seen significant

Depression in Primary Care: Evidence and Practice, ed. Simon Gilbody and Peter Bower. Published by Cambridge University Press. © Cambridge University Press 2011.

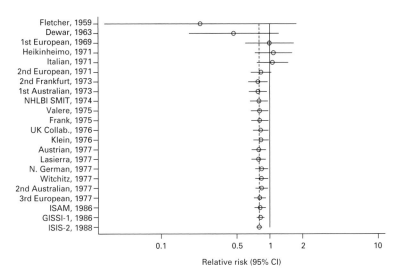

Figure 10.1 Cumulative meta-analysis of 22 trials of streptokinase versus placebo following myocardial infarction.

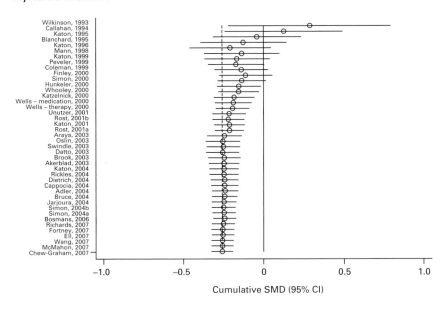

Figure 10.2 Cumulative meta-analysis of collaborative care studies. SMD, standardized mean difference.

changes in the way that clinicians make decisions. Harrison has identified four main models (see Figure 10.3), which differ on two dimensions: whether knowledge used in clinical practice derives from personal experience or external research, and whether implementation of that knowledge is driven by internal or external forces.[3]

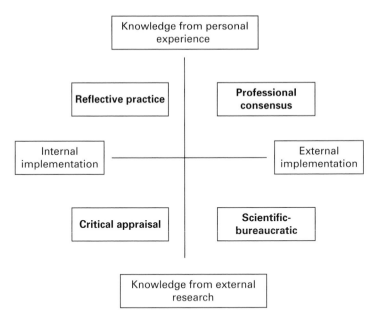

Figure 10.3 Four models of medical practice (adapted from Harrison[3]).

Traditionally, clinicians were expected to use a reflective practice model, with little obvious link to external research or external pressures encouraging change. Criticisms of the limitations of such personal reflection led to a greater emphasis on the role of professional bodies to drive change, which at least avoided some of the idiosyncrasies of personal reflection, but had weaknesses of its own, summed up by the acronym GOBSAT ('good old boys sat at a table'), which highlighted the problems of transparency and professional protectionism inherent in the professional consensus approach.

The rise of evidence-based practice strengthened the role of external research, which in turn led to the rise of interest in the critical appraisal model. Critical appraisal involves health professionals making sense of and applying evidence in the case of individual patients, seeking out evidence to drive their clinical decision making. However, that model was soon seen as unsustainable, because of the limited time available to health professionals and the ever-increasing amount of research available relevant to their clinical decisions.[4] This led to the scientific-bureaucratic model, where professionals take their lead from external research, driven by external bodies. This model is best characterized by the use of clinical guidelines.

As noted in Chapter 2, clinical guidelines are 'systematically developed statements to assist practitioner and patient decisions about appropriate health care for specific clinical circumstances'.[5] Implicit in the guideline movement was the idea that gathering and codifying the evidence was likely to be necessary and sufficient for changes in clinical behaviour. However, evidence from a variety of sources suggests that, although guidelines can impact on behaviour, their impact is generally quite limited.[6,7] Partly, this reflects the relative simplicity of the model on which guidelines are based, which assumes that a lack of knowledge is the primary cause of problems in quality of care, and ignores the many factors that can impact on the success or otherwise of attempts to change clinical behaviour. For example, the failure of healthcare workers to engage in practices to enhance hand hygiene reflects influences at different levels of the care system (e.g. individual professional, clinical teams and organizations) and can be explained using a variety of theories. These include cognitive theories relating to knowledge, behavioural theories relating to cues in the environment, social influence theories involving social norms and the effects of the wider group, and organizational theories that highlight the wider system in which the professional operates.[4]

There is now a realization that as well as the need for a science and technology to underpin evidence-based practice, there is a need for a complementary science and technology concerning the *translation* of evidence into practice, if the potential of evidence-based practice is to be realized in terms of changes in patient health and well-being. This chapter will outline some of the developments in that area and consider how they apply to the problems of depression care.

Definitions

The science of knowledge translation is a relatively new one, and definitions are changing rapidly.[8] Broadly speaking, it is possible to distinguish three different types of 'translation', differentiated by levels of activity and scope. *Diffusion* has been defined as the passive spread of innovations, whereas more active approaches may be defined as *dissemination* (i.e. 'the targeted distribution of information and intervention materials to a specific public health or clinical practice audience' with 'the intent to spread knowledge and the associated evidence-based interventions') or *implementation* ('the use of strategies to introduce or change evidence-based health interventions within specific settings').[8,9] Good clinical practice developed locally and spread through informal professional contacts might represent an example of diffusion, whereas sending out written clinical guidelines to practitioners would be an example of dissemination. Finally, actively engaging with practices to help them change their clinical practice in line with those guidelines and implement a new model of care would be an example of implementation.

Models of translation

The present book is structured around different models of quality improvement in depression. Increasingly, it is recognized that there is a need for models of translation. At present, there is no consensus about the optimal way to understand the process of translation: indeed, a recent review highlighted the many ways in which the diffusion of knowledge can be understood.[10] We will outline exemplar models, to illustrate the factors that can determine the success of efforts to change care delivery. We will finish by exploring the relevance of these models in the specific area of the care of depression.

The development of evidence-based intervention strategies is only one step towards the translation of that benefit for population health. Instead, evidence must be married to effective implementation strategies, which themselves have to be considered at multiple levels (e.g. systems, organizations, groups and individuals). Traditional guideline implementation has assumed that changes in clinical behaviour can be understood at the level of individual decision making, and has tended to ignore the other levels.

Translation strategies also have their own outcomes. These include *fidelity* (the degree to which the intervention as designed is delivered in practice), *acceptability* (in terms of the views of the professionals being targeted by implementation activities) and *penetration* (the proportion of health professionals taking up the intervention). It is only when these outcomes have been achieved successfully that evidence-based interventions may start to impact on care processes and patient outcomes.[8]

A relevant model is the PARIHS framework (Promoting Action on Research Implementation in Health Services – www.parihs.org).[11,12] The PARIHS framework is designed to describe the optimal conditions under which translation is likely to be successful. The model describes three key issues:

- *Evidence*: this comprises a number of forms of evidence, of which research evidence of the type summarized in this book is only one. Other types include clinical experience, patient preferences and local information. Each of these types of evidence can be considered to have strong and weak forms. For example, rigorous evidence is preferable to less rigorous designs, while greater weight is placed on clinical experience that has been through a process of reflection, critique and debate, compared with that based on tradition.
- *Context*: contextual factors fall under three core headings of culture, leadership and evaluation. Culture refers to the degree to which an organization can be described as a 'learning organization' conducive to facilitating change. Leadership refers to the ability of leaders to inspire a shared vision in a way that is enabling, and which in turn assists in the development of effective teamwork and organization. Evaluation refers to the ability of the organization to generate evidence concerning the success or otherwise of change for the purposes of feedback.
- *Facilitation*: a facilitator is someone who makes change easier for an organization or an individual. Facilitation can be distinguished according to *purpose* (i.e. focused on specific tasks or more global reflection), *role* (ranging from 'hands on' change management or more diffuse learning and counselling) and *skills and attributes* (the range and flexibility available to the facilitator).

The PARIHS framework suggests that favourable context and evidence both make successful translation more likely (see Figure 10.4). Problems in context can be overcome through facilitation, but different types of facilitation may be required with different combinations of context and evidence.[11]

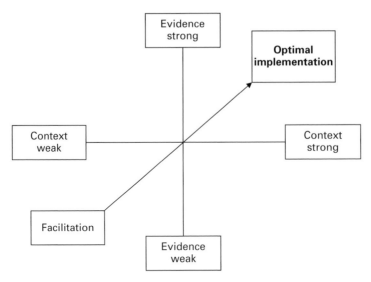

Figure 10.4 PARIHS framework for implementation (adapted from www.parihs.org).[11,12]

Translation of evidence in depression care

The previous section has outlined some of the models that have been used to make sense of knowledge translation in health services in general. How do these apply in the specific case of depression?

Effective translation means understanding the different levels impacting on the process. The critical levels of change in depression care have been outlined.[13] At the level of the individual patient and the wider community, key issues include knowledge about mental health in general and depression in particular, preferences about care, and the important issue of attitudes towards mental health and associated stigma. Among the psychological factors likely to account for failures of depression care are: lack of awareness; lack of familiarity; lack of agreement; lack of self efficacy; lack of outcome expectancy; and the inertia of previous practice.[14]

The next level has been described as the 'microsystem of care', and refers to the work conducted in clinics by doctors, nurses and other health professionals. Here, important drivers include the structure of care (which may be designed to deal with acute problems, or focused on physical illness), available technology and other resources, and the critical issue of the limited time available to health professionals.[15]

At the level of the organization (for example, the individual general practice or family practice clinic, or the health plan), there are issues concerning the priority given to quality improvement, associated incentives, as well as issues of leadership.[13] Finally, there is the issue of the wider environment, which includes the regulatory environment and the various payment systems in place to deal with health professional reimbursement and the costs of care. Chapter 11 highlights the role of financial incentives in encouraging adoption of certain clinical practices of relevance to depression in the UK.[16,17]

Translation becomes difficult because of these multiple levels, which may not be aligned. For example, providing the technology, resources and time to provide depression care may not be sufficient if the incentives are not in place to encourage behaviour change. Indeed, incentives can serve to make the desired behaviours unlikely. For example, in the USA, payment systems such as capitation (i.e. payment on the basis of the number of patients in a practice) may incentivize short visits that may not be conducive to high-quality depression care, even if the relevant systems and resources (such as clinical information systems and outcome measurement) are in place.[18]

What does the PARIHS model suggest concerning the difficulties of translating evidence into practice? In terms of evidence, one of the core types required for new models of depression care to be implemented concerns economic evidence. Current economic analyses focus on cost-effectiveness and cost utility, seeking to estimate how much cost is incurred to achieve the benefits of a new treatment or intervention (see Chapter 3). Many new ways of delivering services increase costs, but from an evidence-based practice perspective this may be worthwhile if the increased costs are associated with additional health gain according to some arbitrary but agreed criterion.

However, there is a tension between the evidence-based perspective derived from that of an economist involved in cost-effectiveness calculations, and that taken by service managers and planners, who are focused on cost offset, i.e. potential reductions in costs associated with care.[18] Many innovations fail because a demonstration of cost-effectiveness (as defined in Chapter 3 and summarized in Chapters 5, 6, 7 and 8) either requires additional costs to implement, which may not be forthcoming, or because any cost savings or other benefits fall on other sectors (e.g. employment, housing) that are not to the benefit of those paying for the health service. In this case, the decision maker may not have either the resources or the motivation to implement the change. As highlighted in Chapter 11, one of the main drivers for improvements in mental healthcare in the UK is the work of the economist Richard Layard, who made a case for cost offset from mental healthcare to support his proposals.[19]

A number of studies in depression have highlighted the importance of leadership.[20] There is a need to engage leaders at all levels of the organization, to ensure that development is seen as a useful tool, not simply another requirement.[21] Leadership 'buy in' can be used to justify behaviour change, to motivate colleagues and to provide fiscal and other incentives, while also providing knowledge of the wider environment and wider group of stakeholders who might be effected.[22] Turnover of leaders has been identified as a predictor of failure to sustain the Chronic Care Model on which the collaborative care model is based.[22] Again, in the UK, it was both the intellectual case made by Layard combined with his leadership influence at the highest levels of government that contributed to change, as the intellectual case had been made many times before to little avail.[23,24]

Another impact of context relates to the issue of standardization and customization. There is a tension in the translation literature concerning the advantages and disadvantages of customizing models to the needs of particular environments and clinical organizations. For example, it has been suggested that in the case of collaborative care, large sites might wish to have dedicated nurse care managers, whereas in small sites, one person might take up the role as part of their work.[21] Alternatively, consultation-liaison might be delivered differently in rural and urban settings, with greater use of telepsychiatry interventions (i.e. delivery of mental health services through telecommunications and information technology) in the former to assist in arranging liaison meetings between dispersed professionals. However, there is the issue of implementation fidelity to consider. The evidence may relate to a specific way of delivering depression care, and fidelity to that way of delivery may be associated with outcome, which cautions against excessive amounts of customization. For example, acting as a case manager for part of the working week may lead to tensions between that role and other roles, which may impact on the effectiveness of the intervention. Similarly, although telemedicine may be more feasible and acceptable for arranging liaison meetings, the technology may mean that the benefits of the meetings are attenuated. This loss of effectiveness following customization has been characterized as a 'voltage drop',[25] and is a real tension in translation research.

Finally, the role of evaluation is important. Innovators in the UK used to faced significant barriers in encouraging the use of routine outcome measurement in the evaluation of mental health services, for a variety of reasons including clinical inertia, inexperience and antipathy to the use of objective outcome measures.[26] However, once those barriers had been overcome (in part through linking them to the introduction of new funds and the implementation of 'demonstration sites' – see Chapter 11), then the data provided an objective basis for decisions about the adoption of different service models.[27]

A facilitator is someone who makes change easier for an organization or an individual. Facilitation can be distinguished according to purpose (i.e. focused on specific tasks or more global reflection), role (ranging from 'hands on' change management or more diffuse learning and counselling) and skills and attributes (the range and flexibility available to the facilitator). There has been correspondingly little work on the role of facilitation in depression, although the role has been used in the UK, and a trial indicated that practice-level facilitation (based on audit, education and feedback) may have an impact on recognition of depression, although there was less evidence of an effect on depression care or patient outcome.[28] Recent work on the role of facilitation has highlighted some of the important functions of external facilitators, including problem solving and support, but there is a large amount of work that remains to be done to understand this important dimension of the model.[29] Some of these functions have been implemented through a 'quality improvement collaborative' approach where a number of sites work together to share experience of implementation over a period of time.[30]

Concluding comments

The science of implementation is in its infancy,[4] although the evidence base is growing rapidly. Some core findings about the effective ingredients of change are beginning to emerge, but at present the main conclusion is that implementation is a complex and difficult affair, and producing the evidence only the first step in a long process before the fruits of evidence-based practice can impact on patient outcomes.

REFERENCES

1 Institute of Medicine. *Crossing the Quality Chasm: A New Health System for the 21st Century*. Washington, DC: National Academy Press, 2001.

2 Cooksey D. *A Review of UK Health Research Funding*. London: HMSO, 2006.

3 Harrison S. New Labour, modernisation and the medical labour process. *Journal of Social Policy* 2002;31:465–85.

4 Grol R, Grimshaw J. From best evidence to best practice: effective implementation of change in patients' care. *Lancet* 2003;362:1225–30.

5 Field M, Lohr K. *Clinical Practice Guidelines: Directions for a New Program*. Washington, DC: National Academy Press, 1990.

6 Farmer A, Légaré F, Turcot L *et al*. Printed educational materials: effects on professional practice and health care outcomes. *Cochrane Database of Systematic Reviews* 2008;Issue 3: CD004398. DOI: 10.1002/14651858.CD004398.pub2.

7 Kendrick T. Why can't GPs follow guidelines on depression? *British Medical Journal* 2000;320:200–1.

8 Proctor E, Landsverk J, Aarons G, Chambers D, Glisson C, Mittman B. Implementation research in mental health services: an emerging science with conceptual, methodological, and training challenges. *Administration and Policy in Mental Health and Mental Health Services Research* 2009;36:34

9 Greenhalgh T, Robert G, Macfarlane F, Bate P, Kyriakidou O. Diffusion of innovations in service organizations: systematic review and recommendations. *Milbank Quarterly* 2004;82:581–629.

10 Greenhalgh T, Robert G, Macfarlane F, Bate P, Kyriakidou O, Peacock R. Storylines of research in diffusion of innovation: a meta-narrative approach to systematic review. *Social Science and Medicine* 2005;61:417–30.

11 Kitson A, Rycroft-Malone J, Harvey G, McCormack B, Seers K, Titcheno A. Evaluating the successful implementation of evidence into practice using the PARiHS framework: theoretical and practical challenges. *Implementation Science* 2008;3:1.

12 Rycroft-Malone J. The PARIHS framework – a framework for guiding the implementation of evidence based practice. *Journal of Nursing Care Quality* 2009;19:297–304.

13 Katon W. The Institute of Medicine 'Chasm' report: implications for depression collaborative care models. *General Hospital Psychiatry* 2003;25:222–9.

14 Cabana M, Rushton J, Rush J. Implementing practice guidelines for depression: applying a new framework to an old problem. *General Hospital Psychiatry* 2002;24:35–42.

15 Von Korff M, Goldberg D. Improving outcomes in depression. *British Medical Journal* 2001;323:948–9.

16 Dowrick C, Leydon G, McBride A *et al.* Patients' and doctors' views on depression severity questionnaires incentivised in UK quality and outcomes framework: qualitative study. *British Medical Journal* 2009;338:b663

17 Kendrick T, Dowrick C, McBride A *et al.* Management of depression in UK general practice in relation to scores on depression severity questionnaires: analysis of medical record data. *British Medical Journal* 2009;338:b750

18 Frank R, Huskamp H, Pincus H. Aligning incentives in the treatment of depression in primary care with evidence-based practice. *Psychiatric Services* 2003;54:682–7.

19 Layard R. The case for psychological treatment centres. *British Medical Journal* 2006;332:1030–2.

20 Oxman T, Dietrich A, Williams J, Kroenke K. A three component model for reengineering systems for the treatment of depression in primary care. *Psychosomatics* 2002;43:441–50.

21 Meresman J, Hunkeler E, Hargreaves W *et al.* A case report: implementing a nurse telecare program for treating depression in primary care. *Psychiatric Quarterly* 2003;74:61–73.

22 Kilbourne A, Schulberg H, Post E, Rollman B, Belnap B, Pincus H. Translating evidence-based depression management services to community-based primary care practices. *The Milbank Quarterly* 2004;82:631–59.

23 Friedli K, King M. Counselling in general practice – a review. *Primary Care Psychiatry* 1996;2:205–16.

24 Simpson S, Corney R, Fitzgerald P. Counselling provision, prescribing and referral rates in a general practice setting. *Primary Care Psychiatry* 2003;8:115–19.

25 Oxman T, Dietrich A, Schulberg H. The depression care manager and mental health specialist as collaborators within primary care. *American Journal of Geriatric Psychiatry* 2003;11:507–16.

26 Bower P, Gilbody S, Barkham M. Making decisions about patient progress: the application of routine outcome measurement in stepped care psychological therapy services. *Primary Care Mental Health* 2006;4:21–8.

27 Clark D, Layard R, Smithies R, Richards D, Suckling R, Wright B. Improving access to psychological therapy: Initial evaluation of two UK demonstration sites. *Behaviour Research and Therapy* 2009;1:910–20.

28 Bashir K, Blizard B, Bosanquet A, Bosanquet N, Mann A, Jenkins R. The evaluation of a mental health facilitator in general practice: effects on recognition, management, and outcome of mental illness. *British Journal of General Practice* 2000;50:626–9.

29 Stetler C, Legro M, Rycroft-Malone J *et al.* Role of 'external facilitation' in implementation of research findings: a qualitative evaluation of facilitation experiences in the Veterans Health Administration. *Implementation Science* 2006;1: 23.

30 Fletcher J, Gavin M, Harkness E, Gask L. A collaborative approach to embedding graduate primary care mental health workers in the UK National Health Service. *Health and Social Care in the Community* 2008;16:451–9.

11

United Kingdom perspective

David Richards

Despite extensive reform of the health and social care sectors in the UK in recent years, the general practitioner (GP) remains at the centre of an individualized medical model of care provision. Almost all GPs in the UK are subcontractors rather than salaried workers. Groups of GPs run their own business and are reimbursed for their activities via a complex web of incentives and payments. The extent to which health policy makers and managers can direct GP behaviour is dependent on the extent to which they can manipulate these incentives. The latest and most assertive manifestation of this incentive approach is the 'Quality and Outcomes Framework' initiated in 2004, whereby GPs are directly paid for hitting certain performance targets.[1]

Although the prevalence of depression is high (outlined in Chapter 1), 70–80% of spending in mental health in the UK is undertaken by specialist healthcare providers to deliver care for people with serious mental health problems such as psychosis.[2] Given the epidemiology and the burden of depression compared with psychosis,[3] this leaves very large numbers of people with little mental healthcare. As a consequence of this funding imbalance, the UK's primary care services have traditionally failed to provide an accessible and equitable service for depression, beyond antidepressant therapy.

This has been a source of discomfort among clinicians and policy makers, and various reforms have been attempted to improve the situation, through changes to the structure and delivery of care. The evolution of models of depression care in the UK maps onto the different models outlined in Chapter 2 of this book. This evolution is traced below.

The development of models of care for depression in primary care

An influential piece on the management of mental health problems in the UK in 1966 suggested that:

Depression in Primary Care: Evidence and Practice, ed. Simon Gilbody and Peter Bower. Published by Cambridge University Press. © Cambridge University Press 2011.

Administrative and medical logic alike therefore suggest that the cardinal requirement for improvement of the mental health services … is not a large expansion and proliferation of psychiatric agencies, but rather a strengthening of the family doctor in his therapeutic role.[4]

Although there were isolated examples of consultation-liaison services and the delivery of psychological therapy in primary care,[5,6] the main policy interest remained in improving the abilities of the GP and the wider primary care team, fuelled by a slew of research indicating that the recognition and diagnosis of depression in primary care was suboptimal. [7,8]

This focus on the education and training model found its clearest expression in the Defeat Depression campaign, a multifaceted approach to improving the management of depression through professional training and public education campaigns. Although aspects of the campaign were judged a success,[9] one of the key evaluations was the Hampshire Depression Project, which sought to take the education and training provided for GPs and primary care staff and subject it to a rigorous randomized evaluation. The results (summarized in Chapter 5) were disappointing, with little evidence of any impact on outcome.[10]

The negative results of the evaluation were a blow to the primacy of the education and training model, but there were other pressures. On the one hand, GPs and other primary care specialists have a biopsychosocial focus which means that, for many, the management of mental health problems such as depression is seen to be within their remit. On the other hand, these staff are also generalists, which means that mental health is one problem among many that they deal with, and many staff do not have a specialist interest in this area, nor the desire to develop one.[11]

It was partly on the basis of professional pressures that psychological therapy and the referral model gained prominence, encouraged by changes in financial systems that allowed GPs to employ psychological therapists.[12,13] However, this in turn led to concerns over quality and regulation, and the rise of the evidence-based practice movement also put pressure on these services to prove their effectiveness and cost effectiveness.[14] Several evaluations followed, and although they were broadly positive (see Chapter 8), the limitations of the model in terms of access and equity also became apparent.

Dissatisfaction with the education and training and referral models sparked an interest in alternatives, and it was at this time that literature was beginning to come out of the USA on the collaborative care model (see Chapter 7). The rest of this chapter will outline the recent developments impacting on the models in the UK, and the core issues that will shape the future.

Education and training in the new regulatory and financial context

The education and training model has always suffered from the paradox that effective training is unfeasible (because it is too complex, and only a small proportion of

> **Box 11.1** Clinical indicators in the Quality and Outcomes Framework for depression
>
> **DEP1**: The percentage of patients on the diabetes register and/or the coronary heart disease register for whom case finding for depression has been undertaken on one occasion during the previous 15 months using two standard screening questions.
> **DEP2**: In those patients with a new diagnosis of depression, recorded between the preceding 1 April to 31 March, the percentage of patients who have had an assessment of the severity at the outset of treatment using an assessment tool validated for use in primary care.

practitioners are interested enough in mental health to volunteer), while feasible training is ineffective (because the sort of education and training events that practitioners will attend do not change behaviour). However, as outlined in Chapter 10, context is an important driver of change, and there have been important changes in the context of service delivery in primary care since the failed Hampshire Depression Project.

The first change is the increasing policy emphasis on guidelines, and the development of structures to more explicitly encourage their implementation, culminating in the formation of the National Institute for Health and Clinical Excellence (NICE, www.nice.org.uk).

NICE produced its first guidelines for depression in late 2004, and all mental health care providers are expected to show how they plan to be compliant with the recommendations. Although there is no direct evidence that the NICE depression guidelines have made an impact on depression services, it can be argued that their publication has spawned two of the most significant developments in primary care mental health in the UK to date: the Layard project on Improving Access to Psychological Therapies (IAPT) and the incorporation of the concept of 'stepped care' into mainstream mental health policy – both described in detail later in this chapter.

The introduction of the Quality and Outcomes Framework of the new GP contract was the second major change that gave new impetus to models of education and training. The Quality and Outcomes Framework led to GPs being financially rewarded for achieving a range of quality indicators. Although depression was slow to be adopted within this scheme, GPs were soon being incentivized to screen for depression in certain patient groups (especially those with long-term conditions) and to use routine outcome measures to assess change (see Box 11.1).

Recent research has shown that these financial incentives have had a major impact, with the majority of GPs using screening measures with patients. However, the initiative is an interesting test case for the use of financial incentives in depression care, as there is evidence that the actual delivery of these screening interventions has often been more within the letter than the spirit of the contract. For example, there is evidence that the measures do not have a major impact on clinical decision making,[15] and that professionals are often using these measures without any great faith that they are valid.[16]

However, it is not clear how this will develop in future. Later iterations of the incentives may raise the bar in terms of what is required for financial reward, and there is evidence that patients are positive about some of the changes, which means that initial unenthusiastic adoption of screening among professionals may change if patients can drive service improvement. As noted earlier, one of the factors driving change within the PARIHS framework is culture change, and attitudes may change if the incentives achieve regular use of screening measures.

The development of the collaborative care model in the UK

Compared with the USA, collaborative care has rarely been implemented in the UK. Four early studies used versions of collaborative care,[17–20] but left out many important components, such as recruitment by screening, case managers having a specific mental health background, and provision of regular supervision for case managers (see Chapters 2 and 7).

After a gap of several years, three new trials reported recently in the UK. One pilot trial of collaborative care for adult depression included specially trained case managers and scheduled supervision and found a medium to large effect size.[21] A second trial in London[22] confirmed the utility of using paraprofessional workers (without significant specialist training in mental health) by finding a similar magnitude of effect. A third trial that studied depression in older people[23] found a very large impact on depressive symptoms. The results of these three trials have led to a major definitive trial to test the effectiveness of this model in the UK.[24]

The development of the referral model in the UK

The development of the referral model and the provision of psychological therapies for depression in primary care received a major boost through the work of the economist Richard Layard.[25] Following the publication of the NICE guidelines for depression, Layard persuaded the Labour Government to make a commitment to increase the availability of cognitive-behavioural therapy. Layard's contention, outlined in his subsequent and influential *Depression Report*[26] was that the UK spends more money on social security benefits because of depression than it spends on alleviating poverty caused by unemployment. He argued that a shift in resources from payments that maintain people out of work to those that provide treatment would pay for itself many times over as people returned to work following successful treatment of depression, a phenomenon described as cost-offset.[27]

Upon re-election, the government initiated a programme of demonstration sites to test out how the UK might increase the availability of cognitive-behavioural therapy for people with depression and other common mental health problems.[28] By design, one of the two main demonstration sites in London adopted a referral model. The other, in a large northern metropolitan borough (Doncaster), was designed as a collaborative care model. This programme is the first in the world to provide a comparative evaluation (albeit non-randomized) of these two organizational models of depression management.

Although the programme and its evaluation are as yet at a preliminary stage, initial data suggest that the collaborative care project was handling a higher volume of cases than the referral model and average waiting times were shorter, as were patient contact times.[29–32] One reason for this is that Doncaster employed paraprofessional case managers to deliver case-managed, low-intensity treatments, whereas the delivery of care in the London site was through more highly qualified psychological therapists. Another major reason was the explicit adoption of a 'stepped care' model alongside collaborative care in Doncaster. The next section will outline the meaning of 'stepped care' in the management of depression.

Stepped care

Chapter 2 highlighted the importance of access to care, and suggested that certain models (such as education and training and consultation-liaison) had greater potential to improve access to care than others. This is because these models change the behaviour of the primary care professional, who is in contact with large numbers of depressed patients, and are not so dependent on the availability of specialist case managers and psychological therapists as the collaborative care and referral models.

However, stepped care is a method of improving access within collaborative care and referral models that require more specialist input. Stepped care is a system of delivering and monitoring treatments so that the most effective yet least resource-intensive treatment is delivered to patients first.[33] Such systems aim to enhance efficiency by providing these less resource-intensive treatments (so-called *low-intensity* or *minimal interventions*) to a proportion of patients in the first instance, before providing higher-intensity treatment to those that do not improve with the first step. Stepped care is the organizational bedrock underpinning the recommendations of the NICE guidelines for depression among others. Although the exact implementation of stepped care varies, it is best seen as the product of two simple principles.[34]

- *The principle of 'least burden'*: effective low-intensity treatments are offered to patients first and high-intensity treatments only offered to patients who are at risk to self or others, have a previous history of treatment failure or do not improve from initial treatment. Low-intensity treatments are short and require less worker input (e.g. exercise and guided self-help). High-intensity treatments require more worker input, for example formal cognitive-behavioural therapy.

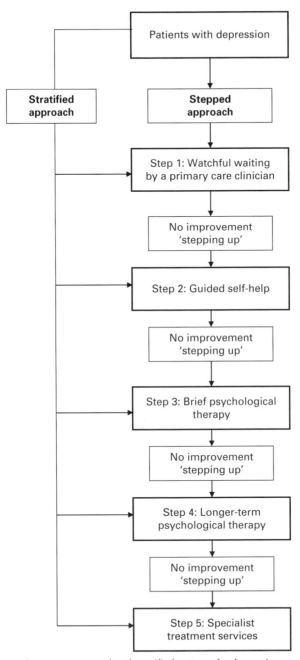

Figure 11.1 Stepped and stratified systems for depression.

- *The principle of 'scheduled review'*: this is required so that patients can step up to more intensive treatments, change to another intervention within the same step or step down to low-intensity interventions including relapse prevention. Reviews should be planned and timetabled, the schedule determined by the phenomenology of the mental health condition, the patient's likely response to treatment and their social situation. Scheduled reviews use objective outcome measures that assist in making treatment decisions.

Despite the simplicity of these principles, the design of stepped care systems can demonstrate considerable diversity. Just as there are four models of depression care described in this book, two models of stepped care can be identified (see Figure 11.1). In one model, patients are initially allocated to interventions at different steps according to objective measures of their symptoms – a *stratified* model. Stratification is often undertaken by a professionally qualified mental health worker acting as a 'gateway' to the service. Alternatively, all patients can be allocated to early steps and stepped up if no improvement is detected at scheduled review – a *stepped* model. The initial steps can be delivered without specialist assessments.

The depression guidelines from NICE are unclear and actually suggest both approaches by designing a complex pyramid of five steps and yet making clear that that many patients will have had treatment at lower steps prior to stepping up.

In practice it is likely that services will design hybrid systems with both stratification and stepping up. Even if a stepped approach is taken, the conditions for making exceptions and allocating patients to higher steps must be made explicit. Equally, a stratified model must still include procedures for stepping people up to higher steps if required. If no stepping up is occurring at all, then stepped care is not really happening. Evidence to choose between the two models is limited.[35]

Concluding comments

There is an argument that mental health in primary care in the UK is poised to make a giant leap forward. Changes to the GP contract incentivizing the recognition of depression, the publication of NICE guidelines and the introduction of the IAPT scheme have come together and reflect a new concern in policy makers for the welfare of those with depression. There remains, however, a potential gulf between rhetoric and reality. Incentivizing screening will not guarantee improved treatment. NICE guidelines have no legislative power. IAPT may only be partially successful. Whatever the international evidence for quality improvement strategies, the individualized, fractured and medically dominated model in the UK primary care setting may make integrated care systems difficult to implement. One cannot deny, however, that there is a chance as we approach the end of the first decade of the twenty-first century that these inhibiting factors will be overcome by the combination of policy maker interest, evidence-based psychological therapy and economic imperatives. It is probably the best opportunity seen to date.

REFERENCES

1 Roland M. Linking physicians' pay to the quality of care. A major experiment in the United Kingdom. *New England Journal of Medicine* 2004;351:1448–54.

2 Peckham S, Exworthy M. *Primary Care in the United Kingdom. Policy, Organisation and Management.* Basingstoke, UK: Palgrave, 2003.

3 Singleton N, Bumpstead R, O'Brien M, Lee A, Meltzer H. *Psychiatric Morbidity Among Adults Living in Private Households, 2000.* London: The Stationary Office, 2001. Available at: www.statistics.gov.uk/downloads/theme_health/psychmorb.pdf (accessed 16 September 2008).

4 Shepherd M, Cooper B, Brown A, Kalton G. *Psychiatric Illness in General Practice.* London: Oxford University Press, 1966.

5 Gask L, Sibbald B, Creed F. Evaluating models of working at the interface between mental health services and primary care. *British Journal of Psychiatry* 1997;170:6–11.

6 Ashurst P. Evaluation of counselling in a general practice setting: preliminary communication. *Journal of the Royal Society of Medicine* 1977;72:657–9.

7 Goldberg D, Steele J, Johnson A, Smith C. Ability of primary care physicians to make accurate ratings of psychiatric symptoms. *Archives of General Psychiatry* 1982;39:829–33.

8 Goldberg D. Filters to care – a model. In: R Jenkins, S Griffiths, editors. *Indicators for Mental Health in the Population.* London: HMSO, 1991;30–7.

9 Priest R, Vize C, Roberts A, Roberts M, Tylee A. Lay people's attitudes to treatment of depression: results of opinion poll for Defeat Depression Campaign just before its launch. *British Medical Journal* 1996;313:858–9.

10 Thompson C, Kinmonth A, Stevens L *et al.* Effects of a clinical practice guideline and practice-based education on detection and outcome of depression in primary care: Hampshire Depression Project randomised controlled trial. *Lancet* 2000;355:185–91.

11 Dowrick C, May C, Richardson M, Bundred P. The biopsychosocial model of general practice: rhetoric or reality? *British Journal of General Practice* 1996;46:105–7.

12 Sibbald B, Addington-Hall J, Brenneman D, Freeling P. *The Role of Counsellors in General Practice.* London: Royal College of General Practitioners, 1996.

13 Sibbald B, Addington-Hall J, Brenneman D, Freeling P. Counsellors in English and Welsh general practices: their nature and distribution. *British Medical Journal* 1993;306:29–33.

14 Wessely S. The rise of counselling and the return of alienism. *British Medical Journal* 1996;313:158–60.

15 Kendrick T, Dowrick C, McBride A *et al.* Management of depression in UK general practice in relation to scores on depression severity questionnaires: analysis of medical record data. *British Medical Journal* 2009;338:b750

16 Dowrick C, Leydon G, McBride A *et al.* Patients' and doctors' views on depression severity questionnaires incentivised in UK quality and outcomes framework: qualitative study. *British Medical Journal* 2009;338:b663

17 Blanchard M, Waterreus A, Mann A. The effect of primary care nurse intervention upon older people screened as depressed. *International Journal of Geriatric Psychiatry* 1995;10:289–98.

18 Mann A, Blizard R, Murray J, Smith J *et al.* An evaluation of practice nurses working with general practitioners to treat people with depression. *British Journal of General Practice* 1998;48:875–9.

19 Peveler R, George C, Kinmonth A, Campbell M, Thompson C. Effect of antidepressant drug counselling and information leaflets on adherence to drug treatment in primary care: randomised controlled trial. *British Medical Journal* 1999;319:612–15.

20 Wilkinson G, Allen P, Marshall E, Walker J, Browne W, Mann A. The role of the practice nurse in the management of depression in general practice: treatment adherence to antidepressant medication. *Psychological Medicine* 1993;23:229–37.

21 Richards D, Lovell K, Gilbody S *et al.* Collaborative care for depression in UK primary care: a randomized controlled trial. *Psychological Medicine* 2008;38:279–87.

22 Pilling S, Leibowitz J, Cape J, Simmons J, Jacobsen P, Nazareth I. Developing an enhanced care model for depression using primary care mental health workers: Implications for the care and management of young men with depression. In: G Baruch, P Fonagy, D Robins, editors. *Reaching the Hard to Reach: Evidence-Based Funding Priorities for Intervention and Research*. London: Wiley Blackwell, 2006.

23 Chew-Graham C, Lovell K, Roberts C *et al.* A randomised controlled trial to test the feasibility of the collaborative care model for the management of depression in the elderly. *British Journal of General Practice* 2007;57:364–70.

24 Richards D, Hughes-Morley A, Hayes R *et al.* Collaborative Depression Trial (CADET): multi-centre randomised controlled trial of collaborative care for depression – study protocol. *BMC Health Services Research* 2009;9:188

25 Layard R. The case for psychological treatment centres. *British Medical Journal* 2006;332:1030–2.

26 The Centre for Economic Performance Mental Health Policy Group. *The Depression Report: A New Deal for Depression and Anxiety Disorders*. London: London School of Economics, 2006. Available at: http://cep.lse.ac.uk/textonly/research/mentalhealth/DEPRESSION_REPORT_LAYARD.pdf (accessed January 2010).

27 Fiedler J, Wright J. *The Medical Offset Effect and Public Health Policy: Mental Health Industry in Transition*. New York: Praeger, 1989.

28 Care Services Improvement Partnership. *Commissioning a Brighter Future. Improving Access to Psychological Therapies*. London: CSIP, 2007.

29 Richards D, Suckling R. Improving access to psychological therapy: The Doncaster demonstration site organisational model. *Clinical Psychology Forum* 2008;181:9–16.

30 Richards D, Suckling R. Response to commentaries on 'Improving access to psychological therapy: the Doncaster demonstration site organisational model'. *Clinical Psychology Forum* 2008;181:47–51.

31 Richards D, Suckling R. Improving access to psychological therapies: Phase IV prospective cohort study. *British Journal of Clinical Psychology* 2009;48: 377–96.

32 Clark D, Layard R, Smithies R, Richards D, Suckling R, Wright B. Improving access to psychological therapy: initial evaluation of two UK demonstration sites. *Behaviour Research and Therapy* 2010;47:910–20.

33 Davison G. Stepped care: doing more with less? *Journal of Consulting and Clinical Psychology* 2000;68:580–5.

34 Bower P, Gilbody S. Stepped care in psychological therapies: access, effectiveness and efficiency: narrative literature review. *British Journal of Psychiatry* 2005; 186:11–17.

35 Van Straten A, Tiemens B, Hakkaart L, Nolen W, Donker M. Stepped care vs. matched care for mood and anxiety disorders: A randomized trial in routine practice. *Acta Psychiatrica Scandinavica* 2006;113:468–76.

12

United States perspective

Stephen Thielke and Jürgen Unützer

The diversity of populations, practices, systems of care and reimbursement models in the USA has set the stage for numerous natural experiments in improving delivery of mental health services in primary care. We will focus not only on controlled research data, but also on efforts to apply different interventions in 'real-world' settings, with an emphasis on organizational feasibility, economic viability and effectiveness.

The current system of mental health service delivery in the USA fails on many levels.[1] Figure 12.1 depicts a general model of how patients with mental health needs receive services. Several types of 'failure' are highlighted:

- many people with mental health needs are never identified (A)[1]
- many of those identified and treated in primary care do not receive effective treatment (C)[2,3]
- many of those referred for specialty care do not receive or continue in it long enough to achieve positive outcomes (D),[1] or do not receive evidence-based treatments (E).

At every step of the process many patients drop out of treatment. The lack of systematic identification and follow-up applies especially to children, older adults, those with low incomes and ethnic minorities.[1] We will address efforts in the USA to remedy the major shortcomings, many of which are at the interface of primary care and specialty mental healthcare.

Screening

Improved case finding through screening (A) and diagnosis and referral (B, D, F) has been a major research focus over the past 30 years. Some controlled studies have shown that screening and systematic feedback of depression diagnoses can increase diagnosis rates in primary care, but this does not substantially effect clinical outcomes.[4] 'Real-world' studies have shown large gaps in identifying patients

Depression in Primary Care: Evidence and Practice, ed. Simon Gilbody and Peter Bower. Published by Cambridge University Press. © Cambridge University Press 2011.

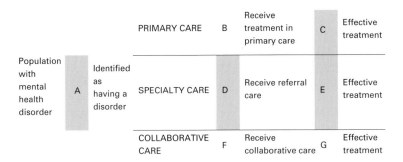

Figure 12.1 A model of delivery of services for depression.

with mental health needs even in systems that nominally emphasize mental health treatment, with at most half of depressed and one-third of anxious patients identified.[5] Untargeted screening of large populations has not shown robust clinical benefits[6] or cost-effectiveness.[7] Thus the US Preventive Services Task Force recommends screening adults for depression in primary care only if systems exist to ensure accurate diagnosis, effective treatment and follow-up.[8] Novel approaches at case finding such as web-based tools[9] and home-based screening[10] have been proposed, but have yet to demonstrate their effectiveness or to be successfully implemented on a large scale.

Provider education and training

Similar to the findings in the UK (Chapter 11), efforts to improve the capacity of primary care professionals to treat mental health disorders through education and treatment guidelines (C) have had limited success in the USA. Even comprehensive and costly training programmes and intensive guideline-based programmes produce only minimal or transient effects on practice styles and outcomes.[11–14] The difficulty of reaching diverse professionals, who already have many demands on their time, adds to the limited feasibility and effectiveness of this undertaking, and systems of care have not developed easily implemented or cost-effective ways of changing practitioner behaviour. Despite this lack of demonstrable benefit, substantial efforts and funds are currently applied to improve depression treatment in primary care in the USA through educating primary care providers in medical school and residency didactics, continuing medical education programmes and organized quality improvement initiatives.

Integrated care

'Integrated care' was initially a term used to describe a mental health practitioner located in a primary care setting and performing a traditional role, offering consultation to primary providers and seeing referrals (combining B and D through consultation-liaison and referral models). Lately the term has been used to describe collaborative care approaches (see below and Chapter 7), but for this chapter we employ this term only in its original usage.

Some primary care clinics have integrated mental health providers into their practices, and some research suggests that such integrated care has better outcomes than traditional care, with similar costs.[15,16] Yet a recent large trial found no significant differences in outcomes between integrated care and 'enhanced specialty referral' (where services were not co-located but referral, transportation and payment were facilitated)[17] despite more patient engagement in the integrated care group.[18] Overall treatment response rates were low in both systems. Some large healthcare systems in the USA (e.g. Kaiser Permanente Northern California, a large group model health maintenance organization serving approximately three million members, and the Veteran's Administration Healthcare System) have integrated behavioural health providers into primary care clinics, but there is little information on the effectiveness of such models.

Specialty referral

Identification and referral of patients with mental health needs (D) represents an extension of traditional service delivery, and has not been the subject of much research in the USA. In some populations, more restricted access to mental health services is associated with higher total healthcare costs,[19] but in other populations additional specialty mental healthcare is more expensive.[20] In the mid 1990s, Callahan and colleagues demonstrated that a programme that identified and referred depressed older adults to mental health specialists was no more effective than care as usual.[21] A more recent multi-site study with depressed older adults in diverse healthcare systems suggests that enhanced referral care may have slightly better clinical outcomes than integrated care,[17] but outcomes in this study were not substantially different from outcomes in 'usual care' practices in diverse healthcare organizations around the country.[22] In general, studies of referral to specialty mental healthcare suggest that rates of engagement with mental health specialists are low, especially for ethnic minorities.[23] Telepsychiatry (defined as 'the delivery of psychiatric services or mental health education at a distance, using telecommunication and information technologies') is a novel approach to the problem of access and specialty consultation, but has yet to demonstrate the capacity to engage or treat large populations effectively.[24]

Collaborative care

Collaborative care interventions for mental health are organized around chronic disease management models (see Chapter 2), and seek to address some of the

Table 12.1 Core processes and roles in collaborative care models

Process	Role	
	Depression care manager	Consulting mental health expert
1. Systematic diagnosis and outcomes tracking	Patient education/self-management support	Caseload consultation for care manager and primary care professional (population-based)
	Close follow-up to make sure patients do not 'fall through the cracks'	Diagnostic consultation on difficult cases
2. Stepped Care	Support medication prescription by the primary care professional	Consultation focused on patients not improving as expected
a. Change treatment according to evidence-based algorithm if patient is not improving	Brief psychological therapy	Recommendations for additional treatment/referral according to evidence-based guidelines
	Facilitate treatment change/referral to mental health as needed	
b. Relapse prevention once patient is improved	Relapse prevention	

systemic failures of traditional forms of care. Unlike traditional and integrated approaches, collaborative care models use 'depression care managers' to educate patients, to involve them in treatment decisions, to monitor outcomes, to ensure follow-up, to support antidepressant medication management initiated by the primary care provider and to coordinate the services of various providers (such as mental health consultation and referral if clinically indicated).

Treatment occurs in primary care, in order to build on the patient's trust with existing providers, to reduce stigma and to improve coordination with medical care. Treatment goals focus on measurable reductions in structured depression rating scales, and stepped care algorithms (see Chapter 11) are used to initiate and modify treatment as suggested by changes in depression severity. The depression care manager collaborates closely with primary care professionals and facilitates the implementation of a stepped care treatment approach that requires changes in treatment if patients are not responding. Care managers are also responsible for tracking a caseload of depressed patients and to prevent patients from dropping out of treatment or being lost to follow-up. A designated mental health expert (usually a psychiatrist) provides caseload supervision, consultation and back-up to primary care providers and depression care managers, focusing on patients who are not improving as expected. Table 12.1 describes core processes and two new provider roles that ground collaborative care.

Multiple studies of collaborative care models have demonstrated their superiority over usual care (see Chapter 8), with advantages in retention in treatment, clinical outcomes, employment rates, functioning, quality of life and suicidal ideation.[25] Collaborative care seems to benefit ethnic minority groups, who otherwise have low rates of care,[26–28] and seems effective for adults, adolescents and older adults with and without co-morbid medical illness.[14,29,30] These are cost-effective programmes[31,32] and they have been found to be effective in a variety of diverse healthcare settings.[33,34]

The challenges of implementing collaborative care programmes include front-loaded costs, mostly from care manager staffing and mental health consultation, and partly from increased adherence to antidepressant medications.[35] Available evidence suggests that such 'up-front' costs may be offset by savings over several years, especially in patients with medical co-morbidities.[22,36] Collaborative care programmes also add a level of complexity to already complex systems of care, and require new roles for and relationships between practitioners and practice staff. The most effective collaborative care programmes involve attention to medication adherence, care managers with adequate training and supervision of care managers by experienced mental health providers such as psychiatrists.[25]

Concluding comments

Findings from 'real-world' experiments in the USA suggest that the best outcomes for treating depression in primary care come from collaborative care programmes that apply chronic disease management models. Such programmes have the best chance of correcting the system-wide deficits that currently offer no or minimal services and follow-up to most people with mental health problems, and they can be adapted successfully to a variety of practice settings and systems of care.

The denominator of an intervention's success should be on a population level, measured by improvements in all individuals identified with mental health needs, and not just those referred or presenting for depression treatment (see discussion of access and equity issues in Chapters 2 and 3). Programmes built around systematic case finding and tracking, patient engagement, outcomes monitoring and stepped care principles that facilitate changes in treatment if patients are not improving will have the best outcomes toward this end. Successful collaborative care interventions have capitalized on information technology to facilitate case tracking and administrative functions. They have developed a team approach in which a care manager, based in or closely affiliated with a primary care practice, collaborates with busy primary care professionals and consulting mental health experts to care for a caseload of depressed patients. Attention to the process of change during implementation of collaborative care, and sharing the results of successful efforts to implement such programmes in diverse primary care settings, should advance our understanding of how to bring such programmes to the people most in need.[37]

REFERENCES

1 Unützer J, Schoenbaum M, Druss B, Katon W. Transforming mental health care at the interface with general medicine: report for the President's Commission. *Psychiatric Services* 2006;57:37–47.

2 Regier D, Narrow W, Rae S, Manderscheid R, Locke B, Goodwin F. The de facto US mental and addictive disorders service system. Epidemiologic catchment area prospective 1-year prevalence rates of disorders and services. *Archives of General Psychiatry* 1993;50:85–94.

3 Young A, Klap R, Sherbourne C, Wells K. The quality of care for depressive and anxiety disorders in the United States. *Archives of General Psychiatry* 2001;58:55–61.

4 Gilbody S, Sheldon T, Wessely S. Should we screen for depression? *British Medical Journal* 2006;332:1027–30.

5 Katon W, Simon G, Russo J et al. Quality of depression care in a population-based sample of patients with diabetes and major depression. *Medical Care* 2004;42:1222–9.

6 Whooley M, Stone B, Soghikian K. Randomized trial of case-finding for depression in elderly primary care patients. *Journal of General Internal Medicine* 2000;15:293–300.

7 Valenstein M, Vijan S, Zeber J, Boehm K, Buttar A. The cost-utility of screening for depression in primary care. *Annals of Internal Medicine* 2001;134:345–60.

8 Pignone M, Gaynes B, Rushton J et al. Screening for depression in adults: a summary of the evidence for the U.S. Preventive Services Task Force. *Annals of Internal Medicine* 2002;136:765–76.

9 Farvolden P, McBride C, Bagby R, Ravitz P. A Web-based screening instrument for depression and anxiety disorders in primary care. *Journal of Medical Internet Research* 2003;5:-e23.

10 Ell K, Unützer J, Aranda M, Sanchez K, Lee P. Routine PHQ-9 depression screening in home health care: depression, prevalence, clinical and treatment characteristics and screening implementation. *Home Health Care Service Quality* 2005;24:1–19.

11 Lin E, Simon G, Katzelnick D, Pearson S. Does physician education on depression management improve treatment in primary care? *Journal of General Internal Medicine* 2001;16:614–19.

12 Simon G. Evidence review: efficacy and effectiveness of antidepressant treatment in primary care. *General Hospital Psychiatry* 2002;24:213–24.

13 Hodges B, Inch C, Silver I. Improving the psychiatric knowledge, skills and attitudes of primary care physicians, 1950–2000: a review. *American Journal of Psychiatry* 2001;158:1579–86.

14 Harpole L, Williams J, Olsen M et al. Improving depression outcomes in older adults with comorbid medical illness. *General Hospital Psychiatry* 2005;27:4–12.

15 Upshur C. Crossing the divide: primary care and mental health integration. *Administration and Policy in Mental Health* 2005;32:341–55.

16 Yeung A, Kung W, Chung H et al. Integrating psychiatry and primary care improves acceptability to mental health services among Chinese Americans. *General Hopsital Psychiatry* 2004;26:256–60.

17 Krahn D, Bartels S, Coakley E et al. PRISM-E: comparison of integrated care and enhanced specialty referral models in depression outcomes. *Psychiatric Services* 2006;57:946–53.

18 Bartels S, Coakley E, Zubritsky C et al. Improving access to geriatric mental health services: a randomized trial comparing treatment engagement with integrated versus

enhanced referral care for depression, anxiety and at risk alcohol use. *American Journal of Psychiatry* 2004;161:1455–62.

19 Horn S. Limiting access to psychiatric services can increase total health care costs. *Journal of Clinical Psychiatry* 2003;64:23–8.

20 Ettner S, Hermann R, Tang H. Differences between generalists and mental health specialists in the psychiatric treatment of Medicare beneficiaries. *Health Services Research* 1999;34:737–60.

21 Callahan C, Hendrie H, Dittus R, Brater D, Hui S, Tierney W. Improving treatment of late life depression in primary care: a randomized clinical trial. *Journal of the American Geriatrics Society* 1994;42:839–46.

22 Liu C, Hedrick S, Chaney E *et al.* Cost-effectiveness of collaborative care for depression in a primary care veteran population. *Psychiatric Services* 2003;54:698–704.

23 Takeuchi D, Cheung M. Coercive and voluntary referrals: how ethnic minority adults get into mental health treatment. *Ethnicity and Health* 1998;3:149–58.

24 Baer L, Elford D, Cukor P. Telepsychiatry at forty: what have we learned? *Harvard Review of Psychiatry* 1997;5:7–17.

25 Gilbody S, Bower P, Fletcher J, Richards D, Sutton A. Collaborative care for depression: a systematic review and cumulative meta-analysis. *Archives of Internal Medicine* 2006;166:2314–21.

26 Schoenbaum M, Miranda J, Sherbourne C, Duan N, Wells K. Cost-effectiveness of interventions for depressed Latinos. *Journal of Mental Health Policy and Economics* 2004;7:69–76.

27 Simon G, Von Korff M, Ludman E *et al.* Cost-effectiveness of a program to prevent depression relapse in primary care. *Medical Care* 2002;40:941–50.

28 Miranda J, Duan N, Sherbourne C *et al.* Improving care for minorities: can quality improvement interventions improve care and outcomes for depressed minorities? Results of a randomized controlled trial. *Health Services Research* 2003;38: 613–30.

29 Bruce M, Ten Have T, Reynolds C *et al.* Reducing suicidal ideation and depressive symptoms in depressed older primary care patients. *Journal of the American Medical Association* 2004;291:1081–91.

30 Asarnow J, Jaycox L, Duan N *et al.* Effectiveness of a quality improvement intervention for adolescent depression in primary care clinics: a randomized controlled trial. *Journal of the American Medical Association* 2005;293:311–19.

31 Katon W, Schoenbaum M, Fan M *et al.* Cost-effectiveness of improving primary care treatment of late-life depression. *Archives of General Psychiatry* 2005;62: 1313–20.

32 Simon G, Manning W, Katzelnick D, Pearson S, Henk H, Helstad C. Cost-effectiveness of systematic depression treatment for high utilisers of general medical care. *Archives of General Psychiatry* 2001;58:181–7.

33 Dietrich A, Oxman T, Williams J *et al.* Going to scale: re-engineering systems for primary care treatment of depression. *Annals of Family Medicine* 2004;2:301–4.

34 Wells K, Sherbourne C, Schoenbaum M *et al.* Impact of disseminating quality improvement programs for depression in managed primary care: a randomized controlled trial. *Journal of the American Medical Association* 2000;283:212–20.

35 Bachman J, Pincus H, Houtsinger J, Unützer J. Funding mechanisms for depression care management: opportunities and challenges. *General Hospital Psychiatry* 2006;28:278–88.

36 Katon W, Unützer J, Fan M *et al.* Cost-effectiveness and net benefit of enhanced treatment of depression for older adults with diabetes and depression. *Diabetes Care* 2006;29:265–70.

37 Katon W, Unützer J. Collaborative care models for depression: time to move from evidence to practice. *Archives of Internal Medicine* 2010;166:2304–6.

13

Conclusions

Peter Bower and Simon Gilbody

This book demonstrates the application of the principles of evidence-based practice and the techniques of systematic review to the problem of the management of depression in primary care. Although both the principles and the techniques are increasingly accepted, there are many legitimate criticisms of their application in healthcare. After summarizing the evidence presented, this concluding chapter outlines some of the criticisms of the approach adopted in this book. We finish with a consideration of some of the key research issues for the future.

Summary of the evidence

We outlined four models of depression management in primary care (Chapter 2), and presented evidence concerning their clinical and cost-effectiveness. The bulk of the evidence concerning depression management relates to the collaborative care model, and the other models could clearly benefit from more research. Evidence to date suggests that the collaborative care and referral models are the two with consistent evidence of effectiveness compared with usual care. The evidence suggests that the effectiveness of the referral model may be higher, although the imprecision of that estimate and the lack of direct comparisons means that any strong statements in this regard are premature. Economic evidence is limited, but the collaborative care and referral models seem to be associated with increases in costs, at least in the short term. As currently delivered, education and training and consultation-liaison offer few advantages over usual care, and those who manage and deliver primary care services have to face the fact that the promise of more efficient models of care has not been realized, and that effective care for depression may require a significant increase in resources to deliver improvements in outcome.

It should be noted that the evidence reviewed in this book is necessarily partial. We have not considered the effectiveness of antidepressant medication

Depression in Primary Care: Evidence and Practice, ed. Simon Gilbody and Peter Bower. Published by Cambridge University Press. © Cambridge University Press 2011.

per se, restricting our analysis to ways of encouraging the effective delivery of such treatments. The review of evidence relating to the referral model used cognitive-behavioural treatments as an exemplar, although other models were also considered.[1–4] There are many other types of treatments that could be delivered in primary care, such as exercise for depression,[5] that have not been reviewed. There are also other relevant ways of delivering depression treatments, such as preventive treatments,[6,7,8] which might also need to be considered. The interested reader is encouraged to explore more comprehensive evidence reviews such as the UK's National Institute for Health and Clinical Excellence (NICE) guidelines for depression[9] for an indication of the full scope of the evidence and the complexity of summarizing and synthesizing it in an informative and accessible format. The evidence reviews have also highlighted the many limitations in the available evidence, such as the scarcity of economic analyses available for the permutation plots, the absence of significant amount of long-term outcome data (especially outcomes over periods exceeding 12 months), and the absence of data on issues of access, equity and patient-centredness.

Limitations of the evidence

This book is based on the evidence-based practice approach, where decisions about service delivery are generally based on systematic reviews of randomized trial evidence (Chapter 3). There are a number of issues about the utility of this approach, which are outlined below.

The limitations of randomized trials

Despite their many advantages, randomized trials have a number of weaknesses. They are costly and take a long time to deliver results, such that clinical innovations and other developments (such as developments in the delivery of depression treatments using information technology) may have made the interventions tested in trials out of date by the time they have been fully evaluated. There are many situations where trials may be inappropriate,[10,11] such as when significant outcome events (such as suicide) are very rare, or where treatments are strongly influenced by patient preferences. In these cases, other study designs (such as observational research) may be preferable. Trials are not necessarily the best methods for understanding the processes by which depression treatments achieve change.[12] There will always be questions that require other research designs to answer adequately. Although advances have been made in the synthesis and integration of qualitative and quantitative research designs into systematic reviews and in the generation of clinical guidelines,[13] the relative impact of quantitative and qualitative evidence on decisions about service delivery remains a contentious issue. There is an argument that the preferences and needs of patients receive too little emphasis in evidence synthesis. Equally, careful synthesis of scientific evidence of the type explored in this book may be distorted if issues of patient preference are used to make subjective judgements of the relative 'weight' given to aspects of the evidence, undermining the transparent and systematic approach to the evidence that is fundamental to evidence-based practice and systematic review.

'No evidence of effectiveness' versus 'evidence of no effectiveness'

Despite the interest in the management of depression in primary care and the use of systematic review techniques to identify all relevant evidence, the current evidence base in not overwhelming in either scope or quality.[14] There is a danger that decisions about service delivery are premature in this context. Critics of evidence-based practice highlight that limited evidence should be interpreted as 'no evidence of effectiveness', which should lead to a search for more data. However, limited evidence about an intervention is often interpreted as 'evidence of no effectiveness', which leads to the intervention being rejected in practice and also loss of support for further research.[15] The data presented in this book would not suggest that education and training or consultation-liaison should be rejected outright, because both models have only been evaluated in a limited number of trials, and versions of the models may still be created that are effective, especially if there are relevant changes in the wider context of care or technological advances that overcome previous barriers. This is especially important because both models have potential for more efficient delivery of mental healthcare. However, the enthusiasm of funding bodies for such research may be low, especially as there is a weight of negative evidence to overcome.

Internal and external validity

One of the main criticisms of evidence-based practice is that it places undue focus on internal validity (i.e. the quality of methodology underlying the trial), and less on external validity (i.e. the confidence with which a researcher can expect relationships found in the context of one particular trial to generalize to other contexts).[16]

The evidence reviews outlined in this book were deliberately restricted to primary care populations, because of concerns about the external validity of studies conducted in different settings (such as specialist care), and the possibility that the effects demonstrated in different contexts are a poor basis for decisions about the needs of primary care patients.[17,18,19] Other reviews have taken a more inclusive approach, which increases the amount of evidence available to the review, but can have profound effects on the results, and especially comparisons of the relative effectiveness of treatments. For example, the UK's NICE depression guidelines include a significant amount of evidence on cognitive-behavioural therapy from settings other than primary care, while the bulk of the evidence for collaborative care has been delivered in primary care.[9] Comparisons of the two data sets are therefore contentious. There are advantages and disadvantages to both approaches.

However, even this restriction does not remove concerns about external validity. Many of the primary care studies of collaborative care were conducted in the

USA, whereas the bulk of the evidence on the referral model derived from the UK. There is an argument that the differences between these two systems of care are as great as the differences between studies conducted in primary care and specialist settings. Despite the wealth of evidence concerning collaborative care, new studies are still being conducted in the UK to make the case for the model,[20] even though the new studies are unlikely to have a major impact on the overall estimate of effect.

Similarly, even in those studies conducted in primary care, there are concerns about the degree to which patients recruited differ from the wider clinical population.[21] This reflects both the inclusion and exclusion criteria used (e.g. trials may exclude patients with significant co-morbidity), as well as the fact that taking part in trials may be more or less attractive to certain population groups.[22] For example, patients with literacy issues face significant barriers to trials, because participation requires an ability to comprehend written invitations, consent sheets and outcome questionnaires, while certain populations may have attitudes to health research that reflect previous negative experiences.

Another problem with external validity is that it is more difficult to judge than internal validity. Such judgements are always relative (i.e. external validity is always judged in terms of a certain context to which the results are to be generalized, rather than being a defined characteristic of a study).[23] Although many randomized trials and systematic reviews state caveats concerning the degree to which the results can be generalized, it is difficult to make such judgements in a consistent and replicable way, at least compared with technical issues such as concealment of allocation. Little is known about the factors that are relevant and irrelevant in judging the degree to which results will generalize.

External validity can be examined empirically. For example, it is possible to explore the relationship between the effectiveness of treatments and the degree to which they are divorced from routine clinical practice.[2,3] Many trials deliberately seek to maximize external validity, using the 'pragmatic' design approach (see Chapter 3).[24] Such trials use broader inclusion criteria (e.g. including patients with co-morbid anxiety, or alcohol problems) in an explicit attempt to make the trial population as similar as possible to those patients being treated in routine clinical practice. Nevertheless, the very nature of recruitment to trials will tend to act as a barrier to certain types of patients and populations, and there are very likely to be limits to the ability of pragmatic trials to overcome all barriers to recruitment.

Evidence-based practice and practice-based evidence

As noted in the previous section, evidence-based practice highlights the role of rigorous experimental research in assessing the value of treatments, but the artificial nature of experiments means that there will always be concerns about the external validity of the data derived from them, and the degree to which they reflect the sorts of results that might be obtained in the messy and uncontrolled world of clinical practice. Although pragmatic trials are one attempt to overcome external validity issues, a more radical approach is to focus more on the rigorous and comprehensive collection of outcome data from routine service delivery, without any of the technical requirements of randomized controlled trials. Such an approach explicitly prioritizes external validity: the lack of control groups and other protections necessarily weakens internal validity. This approach is often described as *practice-based evidence*.[25,26] Clearly, both approaches have their advantages and disadvantages, and there is debate concerning their relationship in the decision-making process. Some view evidence-based practice as primary – the effectiveness of treatments needs to be determined in a rigorous trial before a treatment can be considered worthwhile evaluating in clinical practice. Once a treatment has been proven in this way, practice-based evidence can be used to explore issues such as the translation of that evidence into practice (see Chapter 10). For example, practice-based evidence can be used to explore variation among services and professionals in their ability to demonstrate the sorts of outcomes that might be expected from the randomized controlled trial evidence. From this perspective, evidence-based practice and practice-based evidence are partners, but not equal ones. However, others view them as complementary, with both having particular advantages and disadvantages in relation to certain issues and particular decision makers.[27] At present, among many decision makers, the former view holds more sway, but attitudes to these issues may change over time.

Clinical and service delivery issues

Why are certain models effective, and others ineffective? One of the criticisms of systematic reviews and randomized trials is that they evaluate the worth of an intervention but are unable to explain the reasons why some work and others do not. Although there are techniques by which such issues can be explored through trials and reviews,[28–31] there is an increasing acceptance that understanding the mechanisms by which interventions work requires a wider range of study designs, especially qualitative research,[32,33] and a greater emphasis on theory.[34,35,36]

The education and training model is based on the assumption that problems in the attitudes and skills of primary care professionals (in both the identification of depression and its management) are a major cause of poor outcomes.[37] It is not clear whether the lack of effectiveness of the education and training model reflects the fact that these assumptions are incorrect, or that the best way of improving identification and management has yet to be identified. There is a growing realization that professional behaviour is complex and influenced by a range of factors,[38,39] and one of the key issues that might limit the impact of the education and training model is that many primary care systems are designed to deliver high-volume care, with multiple patient and professional demands needing to be met in relatively short amounts of time.[40] Limited resources of time and the presence of other competing demands may make it difficult to put new skills into practice, even if they are learned.

Much of the education and training literature is also based on the assumption that problems stem from the failure of clinicians to follow evidence-based medication guidelines and a reluctance among patients to take medication in accordance with the evidence. Resistance to antidepressants among patients reflects a complex set of attitudes and beliefs,[41,42,43] and it is possible that interventions used to date have simply failed to address those in an effective way, being based on an assumption of a deficit in knowledge rather than anything more sophisticated. There is also the problem that changing patient attitudes and behaviour may require specialist skills that are difficult to teach to generalist primary care professionals.

The assumption underlying consultation-liaison is that specialist feedback to primary care staff will assist with their decision making about patient care.[44] The lack of evidence of effect suggests that consultation-liaison may not include enough 'active ingredients'. For example, evidence outside mental health suggests that meetings between professionals and feedback of written reports (both of which may be used in consultation-liaison) may not be particularly effective methods of changing clinical behaviour.[45,46] Interventions that depend on improving primary care professionals' skills may have less impact if those skills are already adequate and the intervention does not provide primary care professionals with more time for patients.

The effects of consultation-liaison may also be influenced by the variability in professional relationships, which may in turn impact on teamworking functions such as shared goals, communication and trust.[47] In any study, there will be a mix of effective and ineffective working relationships, and positive effects of consultation-liaison in some cases may be diluted by the proportion of relationships that are not effective. The short-term nature of randomized trials also means that if effective working relationships take a while to mature, they may not be identified within the restricted context of the trial.

As noted above, the primary care environment is characterized by limited resources of time and multiple competing interests in how that time is used, e.g. between treatment, prevention, relationship building, etc.[48] The models with better evidence of effectiveness in depression (such as collaborative care and referral models) provide additional time and input from another professional in addition to the primary care professional, and this may be a key driver of their effectiveness.

The collaborative care model is the only one where sufficient evidence is available to explore what factors are associated with effectiveness.[28,49] The most important association with effectiveness is the degree to which collaborative care encourages improved use of antidepressants among those with depression. Other factors that drive outcomes are the use of regular and planned supervision of the case manager and the employment of case managers with a specific mental health background. This may reflect the importance of specialist skills. Interestingly, although studies of psychological therapy in the referral model are effective, the addition of psychological therapy to collaborative care is not related to improved outcome. Further research is needed to explore this finding, and to determine the correct role of psychological therapy in this model.

Future research

As noted above, there is clearly still work to be done in expanding and developing the evidence base for the models. However, this next section will briefly discuss other research issues for the future.

Communication and the delivery of services and support are being revolutionized by the Internet and other developments in communication technology, and the delivery of mental healthcare will probably be no exception. There are already developments in this regard, as studies have begun to explore how depression care can be delivered remotely (i.e. psychological therapy delivered via the Internet) and interactively (i.e. treatments delivered via computer and web-based programmes with limited therapist contact).[50,51] These developments have major implications, as they hold out the possibility of providing treatments with equal effectiveness to those delivered by trained professionals, but at a fraction of the cost.[52] However, as noted previously, cost and effectiveness issues must be considered alongside issues of equity and patient-centredness. It is important that access to such treatments is not limited by the 'digital divide' (i.e. inequitable access to technology itself), and that issues of efficiency do not crowd out the need to deliver treatments that meet the relational needs of patients that have traditionally been seen as fundamental to mental healthcare.[53] It is possible that such treatments will be of greatest relevance for populations subgroups such as those with greater affinity for technology, or those whose personality does not necessarily need or desire the professional–patient relationship to be a core part of treatment.[54]

Co-morbidity (the presence of more than one distinct condition in an individual) is highly prevalent,[55] and there are elevated rates of mental health problems in patients with long-term physical conditions such as diabetes, arthritis and coronary heart disease, especially anxiety[56] and depression, with the prevalence of depression within this group twice that in the general population.[57] Patients with conditions such as diabetes and depression are less physically and socially active,[58] less likely to comply with medical care[59] and more likely to experience complications.[60,61,62] The simultaneous presence of depression and long-term physical conditions results in worse health than other combinations of physical diseases.[63]

Modern healthcare is based on a biopsychosocial model that should attend to the physical and psychological needs of patients.[64] However, many services focus on single disorders.[65] Patients may routinely receive care for their long-term condition from one professional, and consult with another for depression. This is potentially inefficient, and threatens continuity and coordination of care. which are supposed to be core characteristics of primary care (see Chapter 1).[66] Although the ways in which long-term physical conditions and depression interact are complex,[67] they also provide the potential for effective treatments. For example, reducing depressive or anxiety symptoms might improve patients' ability to self-manage their long-term physical conditions, which could improve medical outcomes such as HbA1c. Improvements in the outcomes of long-term physical conditions might reduce the depression and anxiety that patients experience because of complications and poor physical health. However, there is also the possibility of clashes between conditions and their treatment. For example, treating depression effectively may see a return of a patient's appetite, which may then clash with effective diabetes care.[68] There are also concerns about the total burden on patients from multiple treatments designed to treat different disorders.[69,70]

Research has already begun to address the potential role of the models outlined in this book in the care of patients with co-morbid physical disorders. The recent guidelines on depression care for patients with long-term conditions in the UK recommended the use of collaborative care in patients with long-term conditions, but not depression in the general population, because of the differing evidence of effect in the two groups.[71] It is not clear whether patients with depression and a long-term physical condition should have their depression treated in the same way as patients with depression alone, or whether specific interventions need to be developed that are sensitized to the needs of these groups and can provide a more acceptable and effective intervention. The management of such problems in a key challenge for the future.

Concluding comments

Evidence-based practice has a number of key limitations, and its effective application requires an understanding of those limitations and their effects on the process of evidence synthesis. Even applying the most rigorous methods in a transparent and consistent way will not entirely remove controversies about the interpretation of findings, and we are unlikely ever to have the amount of evidence we require to make our decision making truly 'evidence based'. Nevertheless, we hope we have shown in this book how decisions about the delivery of healthcare can be informed and improved, for the benefit of patients, professionals and society.

REFERENCES

1 Mynors-Wallis L, Gath D, Day A, Baker F. Randomised controlled trial of problem solving treatment, antidepressant medication, and combined treatment for major depression in primary care. *British Medical Journal* 2000;320:26–30.

2 Ward E, King M, Lloyd M *et al.* Randomised controlled trial of non-directive counselling, cognitive-behaviour therapy and usual GP care for patients with depression. I: Clinical effectiveness. *British Medical Journal* 2000;321:1383–8.

3 Brodaty H, Andrews G. Brief psychotherapy in family practice – a controlled prospective intervention trial. *British Journal of Psychiatry* 1983;143:11–19.

4 Schulberg H, Block M, Madonia M *et al.* Treating major depression in primary care practice: eight month clinical outcomes. *Archives of General Psychiatry* 1996;53: 913–19.

5 Lawlor D, Hopker S. The effectiveness of exercise as an intervention in the management of depression: systematic review and meta-regression analysis of randomised controlled trials. *British Medical Journal* 2001;322:763.

 6 Brown J, Cochrane R, Mack C, Leung N, Hancox T. Comparison of effectiveness of large scale stress workshops with small stress/anxiety management training groups. *Behavioural and Cognitive Psychotherapy* 1998;26:219–35.

 7 Jorm A, Griffiths K, Christensen H, Korten A, Parslow R, Rodgers B. Providing information about the effectiveness of treatment options to depressed people in the community: a randomized controlled trial of effects on mental health literacy, help-seeking and symptoms. *Psychological Medicine* 2003;33:1071–9.

 8 Corney R. The role of counselling in primary prevention. In: T Kendrick, A Tylee, P Freeling, editors. *The Prevention of Mental Illness in Primary Care*. Cambridge: Cambridge University Press, 1997:130–45.

 9 National Institute for Health and Clinical Excellence. *Depression: The Treatment and Management of Depression in Adults (Update)*. London: National Institute for Health and Clinical Excellence, 2009. Available at: www.nice.org.uk/nicemedia/pdf/Depression_ Update_FULL_GUIDELINE.pdf

10 Black N. Why we need observational studies to evaluate the effectiveness of health care. *British Medical Journal* 1996;312:1215–18.

11 Jadad A. *Randomised Controlled Trials: A User's Guide*. London: BMJ Books, 1998.

12 Bower P, King M. Randomised controlled trials and the evaluation of psychological therapy. In: N Rowland, S Goss, editors. *Evidence-Based Counselling and Psychological Therapies*. London: Routledge, 2000;79–110.

13 Dixon-Woods M, Agarwal S, Jones D, Young B, Sutton A. Synthesising qualitative and quantitative evidence: a review of possible methods. *Journal of Health Services Research and Policy* 2005;10:45–53.

14 Guyatt G, Oxman A, Vist E *et al*. GRADE: an emerging consensus on rating quality of evidence and strength of recommendations. *British Medical Journal* 2008;336:924–6.

15 Altman D, Bland M. Absence of evidence is not evidence of absence. *British Medical Journal* 1995;311:485.

16 Campbell D. Relabeling internal and external validity for applied social scientists. In: W Trochim, editor. *Advances in Quasi-Experimental Design and Analysis*. San Francisco, CA: Jossey-Bass, 1986;67–77.

17 Raine R, Haines A, Sensky T, Hutchings A, Larkin K, Black N. Systematic review of mental health interventions for patients with common somatic symptoms: can research evidence from secondary care be extrapolated to primary care? *British Medical Journal* 2002;325:1082.

18 Churchill R, Hunot V, Corney R *et al*. A systematic review of controlled trials of the effectiveness and cost-effectiveness of brief psychological treatments for depression. *Health Technology Assessment* 2001;5:1–173.

19 Cuijpers P, Van Straten A, van Schaik A, Andersson G. Psychological treatment of depression in primary care: a meta-analysis. *British Journal of General Practice* 2009;59:51–60.

20 Richards D, Hughes-Morley A, Hayes R *et al*. Collaborative Depression Trial (CADET): multi-centre randomised controlled trial of collaborative care for depression – study protocol. *BMC Health Services Research* 2009;9:188.

21 Naylor CD. Grey zones of clinical practice: some limits to evidence based medicine. *Lancet* 1995;345:840–2.

22 Ross S, Grant A, Counsell C, Gillespie W, Russell I, Prescott R. Barriers to participation in randomised controlled trials: a systematic review. *Journal of Clinical Epidemiology* 1999;52:1143–56.

23 Shadish W, Navarro A, Crits-Christoph P *et al*. Evidence that therapy works in clinically representative populations. *Journal of Consulting and Clinical Psychology* 1997;65:355–65.

24 Hotopf M, Churchill R, Lewis G. Pragmatic randomised trials in psychiatry. *British Journal of Psychiatry* 1999;175:217–23.

25 Barkham M, Mellor-Clark J. Rigour and relevance: the role of practice-based evidence in the psychological therapies. In: N Rowland, S Goss, editors. *Evidence-Based Counselling and Psychological Therapies*. London: Routledge, 2000;127–44.

26 Barkham M, Mellor-Clark J. Bridging evidence-based practice and practice-based evidence: developing a rigorous and relevant knowledge for the psychological therapies. *Clinical Psychology and Psychotherapy* 2003;10:319–27.

27 Bower P. Efficacy in evidence-based practice. *Clinical Psychology and Psychotherapy* 2003;10:328–36.

28 Bower P, Gilbody S, Richards D, Fletcher J, Sutton A. Collaborative care for depression in primary care. Making sense of a complex intervention: systematic review and meta regression. *British Journal of Psychiatry* 2006;189:484–93.

29 Welton N, Caldwell D, Adamopoulos E, Vedhara K. Mixed treatment comparison metaanalysis of complex interventions: psychological interventions in coronary heart disease. *American Journal of Epidemiology* 2009;169:1158–65.

30 Kraemer H, Wilson G, Fairburn C, Agras W. Mediators and moderators of treatment effects in randomized clinical trials. *Archives of General Psychiatry* 2002;59:877–83.

31 Baron R, Kenny D. The moderator-mediator distinction in social psychological research: conceptual, strategic and statistical considerations. *Journal of Personality and Social Psychology* 1986;51:1173–82.

32 Craig P, Dieppe P, Macintyre S, Michie S, Nazareth I, Petticrew M. Developing and evaluating complex interventions: the new Medical Research Council guidance. *British Medical Journal* 2008;337:a1655.

33 Corrigan M, Cupples M, Smith S *et al*. The contribution of qualitative research in designing a complex intervention for secondary prevention of coronary heart disease in two different healthcare systems. *BMC Health Services Research* 2006;6:90.

34 Campbell M, Fitzpatrick R, Haines A *et al*. Framework for design and evaluation of complex interventions to improve health. *British Medical Journal* 2000;321:694–6.

35 Campbell N, Murray E, Darbyshire J *et al*. Designing and evaluating complex interventions to improve health care. *British Medical Journal* 2007;334:455–9.

36 Craig P, Dieppe P, Macintyre S, Michie S, Nazareth I, Petticrew M. *Developing and Evaluating Complex Interventions: New Guidance*. London: Medical Research Council, 2008. Available at: www.mrc.ac.uk/Utilities/Documentrecord/index.htm?d=MRC004871 (accessed 20 November 2008).

37 Schulberg H, McClelland M. A conceptual model for educating primary care providers in the diagnosis and treatment of depression. *General Hospital Psychiatry* 1987;9:1–10.

38 Grol R. Beliefs and evidence in changing clinical practice. *British Medical Journal* 1997;315:418–21.

39 Grol R, Grimshaw J. From best evidence to best practice: effective implementation of change in patients' care. *Lancet* 2003;362:1225–30.

40 Rost K, Nutting P, Smith J, Coyne J, Cooper-Patrick L, Rubenstein L. The role of competing demands in the treatment provided primary care patients with major depression. *Archives of Family Medicine* 2000;9:150–4.

41 Grime J, Pollock K. Information versus experience: a comparison of an information leaflet on antidepressants with lay experience of treatment. *Patient Education and Counseling* 2004;54:361–8.

42 Khan N, Bower P, Rogers A. Guided self-help in primary care mental health: a meta synthesis of qualitative studies of patient experience. *British Journal of Psychiatry* 2007;191:206–11.

43 Knudsen P, Hansen E, Traulsen J, Eskildsen K. Changes in self-concept while using SSRI antidepressants. *Qualitative Health Research* 2002;12:932–44.

44 Bower P, Gask L. The changing nature of consultation-liaison in primary care: bridging the gap between research and practice. *General Hospital Psychiatry* 2002;24:63–70.

45 Jamtvedt G, Young J, Kristofferson D, O'Brien M, Oxman A. Audit and feedback: effects on professional practice and health care outcomes. *Cochrane Database of Systematic Reviews* 2006;2:CD000259. DOI: 10.1002/14651858.CD000259.pub2.

46 O'Brien M, Rogers S, Jamtvedt G *et al*. Educational outreach visits: effects on professional practice and health care outcomes. *Cochrane Database of Systematic Reviews* 2007;4: CD000409. DOI: 10.1002/14651858.CD000409.pub2.

47 West M, Poulton B. A failure of function: teamwork in primary health care. *Journal of Interprofessional Care* 1997;11:205–16.

48 Stott N, Davis R. The exceptional potential in every primary care consultation. *Journal of the Royal College of General Practitioners* 1979;29:201–5.

49 Gilbody S, Bower P, Fletcher J, Richards D, Sutton A. Collaborative care for depression: a systematic review and cumulative meta-analysis. *Archives of Internal Medicine* 2006;166:2314–21.

50 Kaltenthaler E, Parry G, Beverley C. The clinical and cost-effectiveness of computerised cognitive behaviour therapy (CCBT) for anxiety and depression. *Health Technology Assessment* 2006;10:1–186.

51 Proudfoot J, Ryden C, Everitt B *et al*. Clinical efficacy of computerised cognitive-behavioural therapy for anxiety and depression in primary care: randomised controlled trial. *British Journal of Psychiatry* 2004;185:46–54.

52 Christensen A, Jacobson N. Who (or what) can do psychotherapy: the status and challenge of nonprofessional therapies. *Psychological Science* 1994;5:8–14.

53 Pilgrim D, Rogers A, Bentall R. The centrality of personal relationships in the creation and amelioration of mental health problems: the current interdisciplinary case. *Health* 2009;13:235–54.

54 Ciechanowski P, Walker E, Katon W, Russo J. Attachment theory: a model for health care utilisation and somatization. *Psychosomatic Medicine* 2002;64:660–7.

55 Valderas J, Starfield B, Salisbury C, Sibbald B, Roland M. Defining comorbidity: implications for the understanding and provision of health services and health. *Annals of Family Medicine* 2009;7:357–63.

56 Grigsby A, Anderson R, Freedland K, Clouse R, Lustman P. Prevalence of anxiety in adults with diabetes: a systematic review. *Journal of Psychosomatic Research* 2002;53:1053–60.

57 Anderson RJ, Freedland KE, Clouse RE, Lustman PJ. The prevalence of comorbid depression in adults with diabetes: a meta-analysis. *Diabetes Care* 2001;24:1069–78.

58 Von Korff M, Katon W, Lin E *et al*. Potentially modifiable factors associated with disability among people with diabetes. *Psychosomatic Medicine* 2005;67:233–40.

59 Piette J, Richardson C, Valenstein M. Addressing the needs of patients with multiple chronic illnesses: the case of diabetes and depression. *American Journal of Managed Care* 2004;10:152–62.

60 de Groot M, Anderson R, Freedland K, Clouse R, Lustman P. Association of depression and diabetes complications: a meta-analysis. *Psychosomatic Medicine* 2001;63:619–30.

61 Lustman P, Anderson A, Freedland K, de Groot M, Carney R, Clouse R. Depression and poor glycemic control: a meta-analytic review of the literature. *Diabetes Care* 2000;23:934–42.

62 Anderson R, Grigsby A, Freedland K *et al.* Anxiety and poor glycemic control: a meta-analytic review of the literature. *International Journal of Psychiatry in Medicine* 2002;32:235–47.

63 Moussavi S, Chatterji S, Verdes E, Tandon A, Patel V, Ustun B. Depression, chronic diseases, and decrements in health: results from the World Health Surveys. *Lancet* 2007;370:851–8.

64 Engel G. The need for a new medical model: a challenge for biomedicine. *Science* 1977;196:129–35.

65 Starfield B. Threads and yarns: weaving the tapestry of comorbidity. *Annals of Family Medicine* 2006;4:101–3.

66 Haggerty J, Reid R, Freeman G, Starfield B, Adair C, McKendry R. Continuity of care: a multidisciplinary perspective. *British Medical Journal* 2003;327:1219–21.

67 Golden S, Lazo M, Carnethorn M *et al.* Examining a bidirectional association between depressive symptoms and diabetes. *Journal of the American Medical Association* 2008;299:2751–9.

68 Detweiler-Bedell J, Friedman M, Leventhal H, Miller I, Leventhal E. Integrating co-morbid depression and chronic physical disease management: Identifying and resolving failures in self-regulation. *Clinical Psychology Review* 2008;28:1426–46.

69 Lin E, Katon W, Rutter C *et al.* Effects of enhanced depression treatment on diabetes self-care. *Annals of Family Medicine* 2006;4:46–53.

70 May C, Montori V, Mair F. We need minimally disruptive medicine. *British Medical Journal* 2009;339:b2803

71 National Institute for Health and Clinical Excellence. *Depression in Adults with a Chronic Physical Health Problem: Treatment and Management.* London: National Institute for Health and Clinical Excellence, 2009. Available at: www.nice.org.uk/nicemedia/pdf/CG91FullGuideline.pdf

Index